The Stata Survival
Manual

The Stata Survival Manual

Pevalin and Robson

Open University Press
McGraw-Hill Education
McGraw-Hill House
Shoppenhangers Road
Maidenhead
Berkshire
England
SL6 2QL

email: enquiries@openup.co.uk
world wide web: www.openup.co.uk

and Two Penn Plaza, New York, NY 10121-2289, USA

First published 2009
Reprinted 2010

A catalogue record of this book is available from the British Library

ISBN-13: 978-0-33-522388-6 (pb) 978-0-33-522387-9 (hb)
ISBN-10: 0-33-552388-5 (pb) 0-33-522387-7 (hb)

Library of Congress Cataloging-in-Publication Data
CIP data applied for

Typeset by Graphicraft Limited, Hong Kong
Printed in the UK by CPI Antony Rowe, Chippenham, Wiltshire

The **McGraw-Hill** Companies

Contents

Introduction

This book aims to be a resource for those starting out using Stata for the first time. Thus it is neither an undergraduate nor a graduate level book. This is because we appreciate that at what stage introductions to data analysis and statistical software occur varies considerably by discipline and where it is taught. We anticipate that the main users of this book will be either those using statistical software for the first time (and we think you have made an excellent choice by doing so with Stata!) or those who have used other software packages before but are interested in using Stata instead or in conjunction.

We are aware that, for many, Stata is seen as software that you 'graduate' to after being introduced to data analysis using another package. This may have been true for the earlier versions of Stata when the user interface was less developed, but it is not true now. The often cited advantages to beginners of other software, notably the use of pull-down menus, are moot points now as there are multiple ways of interacting with Stata, making it just as user friendly to beginners as any of the other available statistical software packages.

While we understand the benefits of familiarity that the use of pull-down menus brings to those new to the software, we advocate throughout this book the rapid progression to using do files (command files) because a researcher should be able to retrieve, replicate and explain their data analysis as a matter of course. Rather than lament the decline of writing commands and then batching them (we're not old enough to have used punch cards!) in Unix to the main server – only to find there was an error in line 3 after walking all the way to the computer room to collect your printout – we embrace the ease with which users can rapidly progress with their data analysis with well designed software. As teachers, this enables us to spend more time on the 'whys' rather than the 'hows', and we hope that those we introduce to the software and data analysis will continue to use and develop those skills in research throughout their careers.

This book focuses on the knowledge and techniques needed to manipulate and organize data in preparation for statistical analysis, the techniques for generating statistics and the knowledge needed to interpret the results from those analyses presented by Stata. We provide some brief information about when specific statistical tests are appropriate, but this is far from comprehensive and should not be a substitute for a specialized statistics text. Also, since this book focuses on one particular software package, it is not designed to encompass the whole research process. We could not do justice to the complex decisions required for choosing particular research design and data collection methods and tools. What we do have are recommendations as to further reading on these topics and we share these with you throughout the book.

We also provide 'real world' examples and anecdotes. Dealing with real data is usually a messy business and never as clear-cut as some of the initial illustrations may lead you to believe. If you collect your own data, you are bound to get someone who comes up with an answer you haven't anticipated or coded or even takes apart the questionnaire and staples it back together in the wrong order. If you analyse data collected by others, you will need to spend a good deal of time getting to know the data by reading the documentation and wading through the codebooks. Even then the data may not be as 'clean' as you might like. How can this person be 123 years old? How can this person be married in 1992 and then single in 1993 when there are categories for separated and divorced?

Our illustrations are as generic and broadly applicable as possible using variables that would be recognized in the range of social and behavioural sciences. We aim for the book to be used as an introduction to Stata whatever discipline the user comes from. The statistical techniques we cover and the variables we use in our example data are therefore recognizable to any user. We appreciate that what are common techniques in one discipline are rare in others and what may be considered basic techniques in one are viewed as reasonably sophisticated in another. This leaves us a very fine line to tread, but we hope that the techniques covered in this book will give the new user of Stata confidence to go on to other techniques common in their own discipline. Again, along the way we have recommendations for other books that tackle more specialized subjects with Stata.

When we started writing this book, version 9 was the latest version of Stata but we understood that the release of version 10 was imminent. We have tried to identify how version 10 differs from version 9 in the areas that we cover in this book. Version 10 was released in September 2007 with a number of changes from version 9. We cover this in some detail in Chapter 1. There have also been considerable changes to the graphing functions, as seems to be the case in every release since version 6. The biggest change is the addition of a graph editor that helps you make changes to graphs you have already created rather than going back into the commands. This is a very welcome improvement and is akin to the graph/chart editing abilities in Excel, for those who want a familiar reference point. Along with this are some changes to the pull-down graphics menu which we cover in Chapters 5 and 6.

STRUCTURE OF THIS BOOK

This book contains nine chapters. It is always debatable which order of material is best when the actual process of learning software is non-linear and iterative. We have decided to start with setting up Stata in Chapter 1, because there are a number of options available that will enhance the use of the software. Some of you may decide to stick with the default settings until you become more familiar with the software, and we have allowed for that in our discussion. In Chapter 2 we tackle how you get data into and out of Stata. This ranges from how to enter data yourself, opening existing data files in different formats, to how to get information out of Stata into other common software packages such as Word and Excel. We cover a variety of ways to manipulate variables in Chapter 3, while Chapter 4 focuses on manipulating data files such as when you want to merge two together. Chapters 5 to 8 cover common analytic techniques, starting with univariate, or descriptive, statistics, and then moving on to tables, tests for differences between groups, and finally regression analysis. This follows the general way we teach data analysis: univariate, bivariate, multivariate. In Chapter 9 we demonstrate some ways to present your analysis results by taking you through a worked example from research question to the final set of tables and graphs for a report.

In Chapters 3 to 8, in addition to the examples in the main text, we have a demonstration exercise that takes a simple research question on the factors associated with mental well-being and follows with the stages of analysis that are covered in the respective chapters. We try to give you a flavour of the many different ways you can do analyses in Stata. There is rarely only one way to get the information you want, but most researchers have their preferred methods, so try a few and see what suits you. On the first day of our Stata courses we tell students that we expect them to show us something we didn't know about Stata sometime during the course, which is usually met with surprise. However, no course has failed us yet, even when it was being translated into Serbo-Croat!

FONTS AND THEIR MEANING

To try and distinguish between text, Stata commands, pull-down menus, windows, tabs, variable names and data sets we have used different fonts.

This font is for Stata `commands`.
This font is for Stata `results or output`.
This font is for **pull-down menu paths** which open **dialogue boxes**, some of which have **tabs**, and anything else you might need to click on.

For variable names we have used *italics*.

ASSUMPTIONS ABOUT COMPUTER SKILLS

We assume that users of this book will have reasonable computer skills and be familiar with operating typical Windows and file management functions. In our examples we have used the 2003 versions of Word and Excel, so your use of these programs may be slightly different if you are using the 2007 versions; see your software help files or tutorials for more details.

About the authors

Dr David Pevalin
David is Senior Lecturer in Research Methods in the School of Health and Human Sciences at the University of Essex. He spent some time in the Merchant Navy, the City of London Police and the Royal Hong Kong Police, while also studying part time at the University of Hong Kong, before becoming a full-time student at the University of Calgary (Canada). He returned to the UK in 1999 as Senior Research Officer at the Institute for Social and Economic Research at the University of Essex (UK) and moved to his current post in 2003. He has published papers in the *Journal of Health and Social Behavior, British Journal of Sociology, Journal of the American Academy of Child and Adolescent Psychiatry, Psychological Medicine, Public Health* and *Canadian Journal of Criminology*, co-edited *A Researcher's Guide to the National Statistics Socio-economic Classification* (Sage) with David Rose, and authored research reports for the Department of Work and Pensions, the Health Development Agency and the London Borough of Newham.

Dr Karen Robson
Karen is Assistant Professor in the Department of Sociology at York University, Toronto, Canada, and Associate Senior Research Fellow at the Geary Institute, University College Dublin, Ireland. She studied sociology at the University of Alberta and the University of Calgary (Canada) before becoming Senior Research Officer at the Institute for Social and Economic Research at the University of Essex (UK). In 2004, she returned to Canada to teach undergraduate and postgraduate statistics and research methods in the Department of Sociology at York University. At the time of writing, she has been doing research on youth inequalities in the EU, as part of a Marie Curie Excellence Team (based at the Geary

Institute, University College Dublin). She has published papers in the *Canadian Review of Sociology and Anthropology, European Sociological Review, Race and Ethnic Studies, Research in Social Stratification and Mobility*, and *Public Health*. She has a particular interest in research methods and has co-authored the Canadian edition of *Basics of Social Research: Qualitative and Quantitative Approaches* (Pearson) with Lawrence Neuman and co-edited *Quantifying Theory: Pierre Bourdieu* (Springer) with Chris Sanders. She has also authored research reports for the Department of Health and the Department for Education, Family, and Schools.

Acknowledgements

This book came out of our experiences teaching Stata courses at the University of Essex summer school. We have also used these courses for teaching Stata: to government statistical personnel in Bosnia and Herzegovina through our involvement in a Department for International Development project to help rebuild analytical capacity; to government statistical personnel in Albania; at the Office for National Statistics in the UK; and as part of the Prairie Regional Data School and the Western Statistics Seminar series at the University of Calgary in Canada.

The original Stata courses at the University of Essex summer school (which continue to be taught annually by one or both of us) were developed in association with Dr John Rigg, then also of ISER. John was and remains an inspiration to both of us. He can do everything that is in this book, and more, but without being able to see the computer screen and all that we take for granted.

Many thanks also go to the participants of the courses who graciously pointed out errors in our notes and shared their discoveries with us. We wish to thank the author support program at StataCorp, particularly Bill Rising, who gave us valuable feedback. Also to Nick Buck for permission to use the British Household Panel Surrey (BHPS) data for our examples. As with any project, the list of people who have directly and indirectly influenced its development or our knowledge is long, but for a variety of reasons we would especially like to thank John Ermisch, Maria Iacovou, Stephen Jenkins, and Dick Wanner.

The Publisher would like to acknowledge the lifebelt designs in the chapter headings as the work of Sarah Crosby.

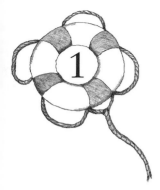

Getting Started with Stata

1

WELCOME TO STATA

So you've decided you want to learn how to use Stata. Great! Whether you're a completely new user to statistical software, or you've been using other packages, we're sure this survival manual will be able to help you with many of the questions you're bound to have.

You've probably come across Stata because your university or employer uses it. Stata has been less popular than its market competitors, such as SPSS and SAS, but is gaining in popularity every year. Stata is now used by medical researchers, biostatisticians, epidemiologists, economists, sociologists, political scientists, geographers, psychologists, social scientists, and other research professionals needing to analyse statistical data. One reason for this is that this software is particularly user-friendly when it comes to analysing complicated data sets, such as those where several data files need to be linked together.

The first version of Stata was released over twenty years ago in 1985. Since then, Stata has changed and developed according to user requests. Like its competitors, Stata is used for analysing quantitative data; but, unlike its competitors, Stata has several features which make it stand out as considerably more desirable. What are these reasons? They will be covered throughout this manual, but we will first turn to some of the resources that are available to Stata users.

RESOURCES

There are considerable resources out there, in addition to this survival manual, to answer questions you might have about Stata. It should be noted that only a minority of these resources are officially tied to StataCorp (the corporation that creates, sells, and distributes the Stata software, along with other products).

Stata website
If you go to www.stata.com you will find yourself at the official StataCorp website. On this site, there is information about StataCorp products, Stata technical support, versions of Stata, and what's new in Stata 'news'. Stata 'news' covers a wide range of topics, including (but not limited to) Stata user group meetings, training courses (such as the ones we teach), publications, and technical updates.

Timberlake website
Another useful website is www.timberlake.co.uk. Timberlake Consultants is a statistical consultancy company that also distributes and sells Stata in the UK. They have a lot of information on Stata on their website, and this is another place to go if you are looking for conferences and specialized training courses.

UCLA Stata 'portal'
The University of California at Los Angeles has a remarkable web 'portal' at http://statcomp.ats.ucla.edu/stata/ which anyone can access. This site is a virtual 'help desk' for statistical and Stata questions that is provided free of charge by the UCLA Academic Technology Service Stata Consulting Group. It is a remarkably rich resource archiving course notes, tutorials, and detailed annotated examples which include Stata commands, the output, and discussion about what the output means. We explicitly draw on some of these resources in Chapter 8.

Statalist
Another resource is Statalist, which is a mass subscriber-based email list. You can sign up for it by going to www.hsph.harvard.edu/statalist and following the instructions. You should note that there is a lot of traffic on this email list and you will get many messages. To give you an idea of just how much communication there is on this list, according to the archives, from 28 February 2007 to 8 March 2007 there were 303 individual messages! And this is just over nine days – you do the maths! There is a digest version available in which emails are batched together, so that you get fewer individual messages in your inbox. There are also Statalist archives (see the website) which you should browse before posting to the list. It is likely that your question has been asked before!

Stata Journal

Stata Journal is a peer-reviewed journal about Stata that is published quarterly. It is available in hard copy and as an electronic version. You can find out more about *Stata Journal* at www.stata-journal.com. The journal contains articles written about Stata as well as user-written software additions. Many of the changes that have occurred throughout the various versions of Stata have been as a result of user input. Some users give feedback to Stata by writing software additions which are programs that do specific tasks that aren't (yet) incorporated into the Stata software. Such user-written programs are often released with subsequent versions of Stata. These additions are profiled in the *Stata Journal* for those who are interested. It may sound like an enormous bore, but we have brought copies of the journal to the classes we teach to show students that the journal is appealing to advanced users and beginners alike. It really is worthwhile taking a look.

Stata help files

Without trying to be ironic, we really want to impress upon you that the Stata help files are really very helpful. If you want to find out about a specific command, going to the **Help** menu and querying a command or searching for a keyword (which will lead to the command you need) provides a lot of information. There are explanations of what specific commands do, as well as the options that go along with each command. Often, there are examples which can help you set up your analysis. Much of the content of help files comes from the Stata user manuals, to which we now turn.

Stata *User's Guide* and reference manuals

If you purchase Stata from a licensed vendor, you have the choice of purchasing the reference manuals at the same time. The *User's Guide*, while a small book, gives you basic introductory information on Stata. A detailed table of contents is found on the Stata website (address above). The reference manuals are a full set of books that, alphabetically, give detailed information about all the commands included in the version you are running (not including user-written additions). The reference manuals are excellent sources of statistical information, as detailed examples often are included, which include annotated discussion of results. There are also subject-specific reference manuals, although these vary by the version of Stata. In Stata 10, the reference manuals include a separate manual on data management, graphics, programming, longitudinal panel data, multivariate statistics, survey data, survival analysis, and time-series analysis. The utility of these books cannot be overstated. If you want to become a regular user, you should have access to a set of these manuals!

HOW IS STATA DIFFERENT?

New and potential users often ask us how Stata is different. Usually, this actually means 'How is Stata different from SPSS?'. As we were both SPSS users for many years before using Stata, we think we can give some straight answers about the differences. But before we do so, it should be noted that, apart from writing this book, the authors have no vested interest in Stata as a product. We are university teachers who have had to learn as well as teach both programs. We both have a strong interest in research methods, and particularly, we both have an interest in answering research questions in the most effective manner possible.

We can tell you that, compared to SPSS, the commands in Stata are much more intuitive and less fussy regarding punctuation. If you fear 'syntax' because of your experiences in SPSS, we are fairly confident that you will find writing command language much less onerous in Stata.

Another strength of Stata is that it is user-driven. When there is a flaw or something that could be improved in the software, Stata listens to its users. In fact, many of the new applications incorporated into newer versions were written originally by users. Related to this point is that Stata, if you are connected to the web and there aren't restrictions on what you can download, is 'web active'. This means that you can download new applications that were written by users to perform specific tasks, and use them as commands. These additional user-written programs cover vast numbers of applications and simply searching for them within Stata and easily downloading and installing these bolt-ons is something that helps Stata stand out.

We both originally moved to using Stata because we were working with large complex data sets and found working with them in SPSS to be very cumbersome. If you have experience of working with longitudinal data sets with various different types of file structures, you will see that dealing with these in Stata is much quicker and easier.

But it isn't the case that SPSS has no strengths over Stata. The editing of output and the labelling of variables, for example, is much easier in SPSS. SPSS users who are used to having a data window open at the same time as running commands will also find it frustrating that this is simply not possible in Stata. For those who prefer to work entirely with pull-down menus, the newer versions of Stata have comprehensive pull-down menus (although we believe that it is a good thing to move on to saveable command files).

Although by no means a complete list of the advantages and disadvantages of Stata and SPSS, it will give you an idea of the reasons why people may or may not change their particular software preference. One of the biggest reasons for not changing is the market dominance of SPSS, although the number of Stata users continues to grow. We personally made the switch when we started working with large and complex data sets – but we haven't looked back!

GETTING STARTED

In this book we assume that you are working with either version 9 or version 10 of Stata, but the graphics we use to accompany the text are done in version 10. We highlight the major differences between versions 9 and 10 later in this chapter. If you have an earlier version, much of what we discuss in this book will be relevant. As this is an introductory book, we will be focusing on the beginnings of data analysis, and these basic functions apply to the earlier versions of Stata as well. We also assume you will be using Windows as your operating system, although Stata can be run on Unix, Macintosh, and Linux.

The first thing you should do when you are getting started with Stata is get acquainted with the various windows that you are presented with when you launch it. Obviously, you need to begin by launching Stata on your computer. Depending on how your computer is set up, this is done by either double-clicking on the Stata icon or selecting **Stata** from the **Programs** menu, which you get to by clicking on **Start** in the left-hand corner of your screen and, then selecting **All Programs**, and then looking for **Stata** in the list of programs.

When you first launch Stata, you may find it off-putting. If you are familiar with other statistical software programs, particularly SPSS, you could think that Stata looks a lot less user-friendly. What are all these boxes? Where are my data? And what's with that black window that looks suspiciously like a DOS screen from way back when? This may instil apprehension if you immediately associate this appearance with DOS programming language. But rest assured, you don't have to be a master of computing languages to use Stata. What we are going to show you is how these windows are customizable, and have features that were introduced as a response to user requests. As soon as you get used to the appearance and set up the windows the way you like them, you will find that Stata is extremely user-friendly indeed. So don't let first impressions put you off.

FLAVOURS OF STATA

Stata comes in four basic 'flavours' – this is their terminology, not ours! The flavours differ according to the size of data sets and numbers of variables they can handle. The first flavour of Stata is Stata/SE, which is especially for large data sets. Stata/SE can handle over 32,000 variables and can fit models including over 10,000 independent variables (we can't imagine a model like this, however). The number of cases or observations it can handle is only limited by the capabilities of the computer on which it is installed. The second flavour of Stata is Stata/MP, which is simply a parallel-processor equivalent of Stata/SE. So if you have a computer with multiple processors and run estimations that take a lot of time on Stata/SE, you have the option of switching to Stata/MP, which is essentially the same but much faster.

The third flavour of Stata is Intercooled Stata, which is the 'standard'. If you are using Stata at a university lab or have purchased a single license, you probably have Intercooled Stata. This flavour can handle over 2000 variables and include just under 800 independent variables in a single model. Like Stata/SE, the number of observations in the data is only limited by the capabilities of your machine.

The fourth flavour is Small Stata, which is very limited compared to the other flavours. Small Stata can only accommodate 99 variables, is limited to 1000 observations, and can only use a maximum of 38 independent variables in an estimation.

What flavour do you have? It will say in the top left-hand corner of Stata when it is launched. For example it could be Intercooled Stata 9.2 which shows that you have main version 9 (updated to 9.2) in Intercooled flavour. Or you may have Stata/IC 10.1 which shows you have main version 10 (10.1) also in Intercooled flavour.

Handwritten margin notes:

1. Stata/SE
   - esp. lrg. data sets
2. Stata/MP
   - same as SE but faster
3. Intercooled Stata
   - 'standard'
4. Small Stata
   - limited

ORGANIZING WINDOWS IN STATA

Stata launches with four windows: Review, Variables, Results and Command. There are considerable differences between versions 9 and 10. Prior to version 9, the window functions were fairly simple and mostly required you to manually change the size and position. In version 9 the windows got substantially more complicated in the default setting with pinning, docking and floating. In version 10 the default window settings returned to simple stretch and drag but with pinning, docking and floating as options. As there are quite a few differences between versions 9 and 10 at start-up, we tackle each in turn.

Version 9

If the four windows (Review, Variables, Results and Command) are not all present, or just for the sake of starting on the same page as us, select from the menus at the top of the screen:

Prefs → Manage preferences → Load preferences → Factory settings

If you follow the above steps, you will get windows that look much like those below. Of course, your 'flavour' might be different (as indicated in the top left-corner), but even if it is, it will look the same upon launching. And obviously, your licensing and serial numbers will be different.

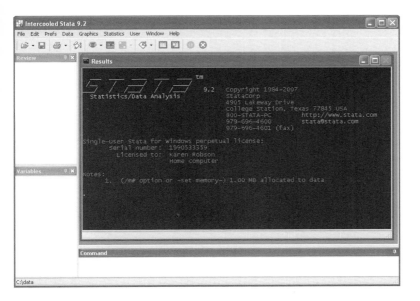

When starting out with version 9 we strongly recommend you disable the pinning, docking and floating functions so that you can avoid problems with windows disappearing or turning into tabs when you didn't intend them to. You can always come back to this later when you want to learn more about changing the display options available to you (see Box 1.1 for more information on this). Select

Prefs → General Preferences

Then click on the **Windowing** tab and uncheck **Use docking guides** and **Enable ability to dock, undock, pin, or tab windows** and then click **Apply**. You will have to restart Stata for the effects to take place.

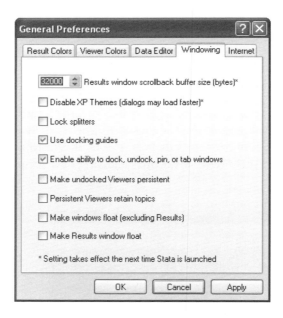

It is possible to resize the windows to suit your own preferences by dragging and stretching them. If you resize your windows, you can select

Prefs → Manage preferences → Save preferences → new preferences set

Then a dialogue box will appear which allows you to 'name' your window settings. This is particularly useful if you share your

computer with another Stata user or if you have different preferences for your windowing for different projects you are
working on. If you relaunch Stata and the window preferences
have changed, provided you have saved your preferences, you
just go to

Prefs → **Manage preferences** → **Load preferences** →
<name of your preferences>

Our preferred window organization is shown below but you can
size the windows, change the background colour, and change
the size, colour and font of the text to whatever you find suits
you best.

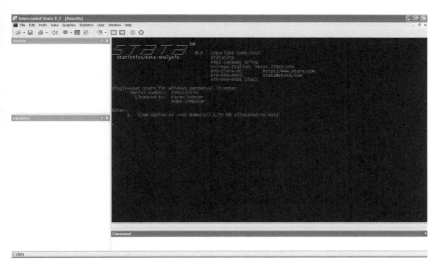

You may choose different settings depending on what you are
using Stata for. For example, you may choose a different set-up
when you are exploring data by mainly using the Command window
compared to the set-up that you prefer when running analyses
from do files. Similarly, if you go on to use Stata for presentations
the windows set-up may be different again. However, we recommend you start with a windows set-up that you like and stick with
it until you become familiar with the software. There's no point
getting tied up in window preferences at the expense of getting to
know the analytical capabilities of Stata. After all, this is the main
purpose of using Stata.

Box 1.1: Pinning, docking and floating windows

Pinning, docking, and floating windows are a default feature in version 9.

Pinning

If you have version 9 and look in the top right-hand corner of the Review, Variables, and Command windows, you will see 🔲🗙. The X symbol closes the window (as in many programs), but the 📌 symbol is used for 'pinning' (hence, it is shaped like a pin). If you click on the 📌 in the Review window, you will see that the Review window vanishes and becomes a tab on the left-hand side. If you click 📌 on the Variables window, it too will become a tab.

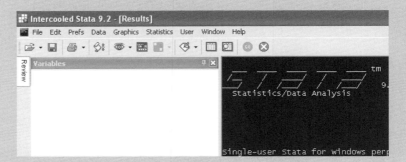

If you click on the tabs for Review and Variables, you will see that they reappear, but quickly vanish once you click in any other Stata window. If you look carefully on the Review and Variables windows when they 'reappear', you will notice that the 📌 symbol has changed to ▭. This sideways position means that the window is not 'pinned'; as soon as you click elsewhere, it will become a tab again.

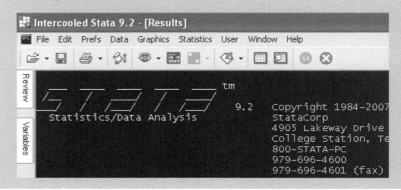

Docking

If you drag the windows around in Stata, some arrows will appear:

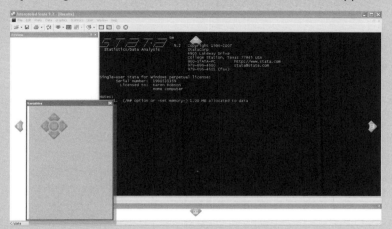

These are docking tools that help you position your windows. If you drag the variables window across the screen – and by dragging we just mean clicking the blue area (in the Variables window in the above screen capture), holding down the left-click button on your mouse, and pulling the box somewhere else on the screen – a number of arrows appear. A compass-like set of arrows has appeared in the middle of the screen and additional arrows appear in at the top, bottom, and right and left sides of the Stata screen. What do these do?

If we select either of the right arrows (either the centre one or the one on the far right), the window repositions as below on the far right-hand side:

▶ You could drag it to different positions, docking it on top, below, or beside the Review window. The best way to familiarize yourself with these functions it to play around with them.

Floating

Windows can 'float' – in other words, only appear on screen when you click on them, and at other times appear as tabs in your Windows task bar. If you double-click on the blue parts of the individual Variables, Review, and Command windows, they will float. They will appear in your task bar and only become visible when you click on them. We have had many students do this by mistake and get very frustrated when they can't get their windows 'back'! All you need to do to restore them to non-floating is click on them so that they reappear in the Stata window, and then *double-click* anywhere on the blue bar of the window to lock them into 'non-floating'.

In version 10 you need to enable these features by ticking the boxes in the *Windowing* tab in the pull-down menu:

Edit → Preferences → General Preferences

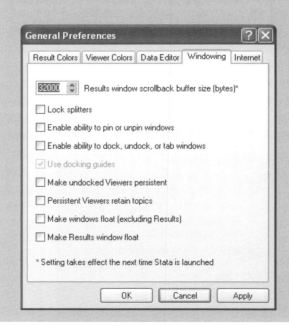

Version 10

Version 10 launches with a windows layout that is the same as when it was last closed. This is fine if you are the only user but if you share a computer with another Stata user, or want to save different layouts for different tasks, then you can save these preferences. To get to the layout you like simply stretch and drag the windows then save your preference using this pull-down menu:

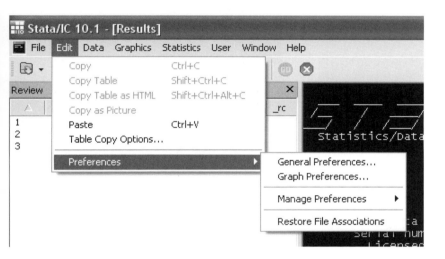

To save your own preferences select:

**Edit → Preferences → Manage preferences →
Save preferences → New preferences set**

Then a dialogue box will pop up which allows you to 'name' your window settings. Then if you launch Stata and the window preferences have changed you just go to

**Edit → Preferences → Manage preferences →
Load preferences → <name of your preferences>**

If you would like to start again with the factory settings follow:

**Edit → Preferences → Manage preferences →
Load preferences → Factory settings**

Our preferred layout is shown below:

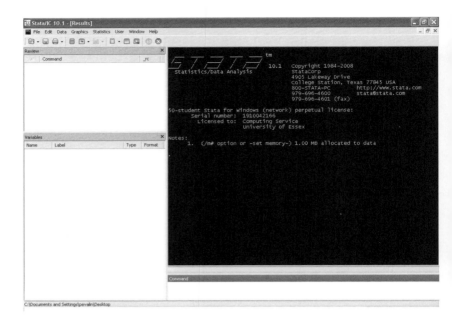

WHERE DID MY WINDOW GO?

Sometimes, by accident, you may close one of the windows on your Stata screen. If, for example, your Variables window 'vanishes', it is quite easy to get it back – just go to the menu at the top of the screen and click

Window → Variables

WINDOWS IN STATA AND WHAT THEY DO

The four windows of Stata that you see upon start-up all have very different purposes.

The Command window
The Command window opens when Stata is launched and is a quick way of running commands, but only if you are familiar with the basic commands. By default, this window is located at the bottom of the Stata screen. We will talk more about typing commands into this window in the next section on 'working interactively with Stata'.

The Review window

The Review window is, by default, positioned in the upper left-hand corner of Stata. All of your commands are recorded here. If you type commands into the Command window, they will appear in the Review window. The Review window is particularly handy when you are exploring your data because if you, for example, do a frequency distribution of a variable, the command will appear in the Review window. All you need to do to repeat the command is either hit the 'page-up' button with the cursor in the Command window or click on the command in the Review window. The command will reappear in the Command window and you can even modify the command (for example, change the name of the variable you are examining) to save on typing. If you double-click on commands in the Review window, Stata will execute them.

In version 10 you can select multiple lines in the Review window by holding down the Shift key and then double-clicking to get them all to run. Also in version 10 you can list the commands in either ascending or descending order by clicking on the **Command** heading. The order changes and this is indicated by the arrow next to the **Command** heading and the numbers next to the commands. A simple illustration of three commands is shown below, first with descending order and then with ascending order.

Review		
	Command ▽	
1	use "C:\Documents and Settings\...	
2	ta d_ghq	
3	su ghqscale	

Review		
	Command △	
3	su ghqscale	
2	ta d_ghq	
1	use "C:\Documents and Settings\...	

Also in version 10, the Review window indicates which commands retuned an error by displaying them in red with the error code on the right. It is possible to sort according to the error codes by clicking on the **_rc** heading. In this way you can easily delete the commands that caused an error if you want to convert your

Review window to a do file. To save the commands in the Review window as a do file simply right-click when one of the commands is selected and you will see an option to **Save Review Contents** which will automatically save them in a do file format.

△	Command	_rc
1	set mem 50m	
2	use "C:\Documents and Settings\pevalin\Desk...	
3	codebook sex age,c	111
4	use "C:\Documents and Settings\pevalin\Desk...	
5	renpfix a	
6	rename age12 age	110
7	codebook sex age,c	

Review ✕

The Variables window

When you have a data set loaded, the variable names and labels appear in this window. Sometimes you need to stretch out the window widthwise to see the variable labels – if the variables are labelled in your particular data set. In version 10 you will see that the type and format of each variable is also listed in the window.

The Results window

In this window, the results of the commands are presented. You should note that Stata does not 'save' the results here indefinitely and that by default, only 32,000 bytes of memory are allocated to the 'buffer'. To permanently save your results you will need to use a log file that we introduce later in this chapter and tackle in more detail in Chapter 2. You can change the buffer to up to 500,000 bytes either by typing in the Command window:

```
set scrollbufsize 100000
```

or by using the pull-down menu:

Prefs → **General Preferences**   (version 9)
Edit → **Preferences** → **General Preferences**   (version 10)

Then click on the **Windowing** tab and at the top you will see the up and down arrows to change the size of the buffer. Whatever size you allocate (between 10,000 and 500,000 bytes) will be remembered by Stata and then become the default every time Stata is launched.

INTERACTING WITH STATA

There are three ways to 'interact' with Stata to tell the program what you would like to do with the data. Here we have called these ways using pull-down menus, 'working interactively', and writing do files.

Before we get on to these different ways of interacting with Stata, it is important that we clarify our terminology. There is a good deal of confusing terminology surrounding the ways to interact – some comes from the language used by Stata, but other users carry over language from other software packages. This can be a little confusing for the beginner. For example, in SPSS the written text files for commands are called 'syntax files' but often referred to as 'code'. The Stata name for a text file of commands is a *do* file, which has a .do extension (see Box 1.2 for other file extensions). That distinguishes it from the SPSS syntax files, but how do you refer to the actual text in the file? Some users carry over the word syntax but we prefer to use commands. So, in a do file we have a series of commands and these commands have options.

Through pull-down menus

If you have used the Windows versions of SPSS then using pull-down menus to manipulate and analyse data will be familiar to you. Version 8 of Stata was the first version to incorporate pull-down menus and, while we strongly recommend the use of do files, the pull-down menus are useful when getting to know Stata, especially for graphing. You will see in the pull-down menus under **Statistics**, for example, a series of options for various types of statistical tests. It should be pointed out early on to the new user that there are more statistical possibilities in Stata than there are options in the pull-down menus which open dialogue boxes. It is not possible to access some types of statistical analyses in the pull-down menus – they must be entered as commands in either a do file or the Command window.

Through the Command window

A second way of using Stata is through writing commands in the Command window and hitting the Enter key. The command then appears in the Review window, and as discussed earlier, can be saved as a do file.

The Command window can be used to directly call up the dialogue boxes in the same way as the pull-down menus use them. For example, typing **db summarize** in the Command window then hitting the Enter key will bring up the dialogue box used by the pull-down menu to produce summary statistics (see Chapter 5 and Box 5.4).

In the Command window the typed commands can run over one line without any problem. However, in a do file if a command runs over one line (or you want to break up the command for ease of editing) then there needs to be a /// at the end of each line except the last. This /// tells Stata to ignore the line break and continue reading the command as if on a single line. We use this /// notation in this manual when our commands run over a single line. If you are using the Command window to follow or adapt these commands, then you can ignore the continuation notation ///.

Through the construction of do files

Instead of just typing commands into the Command window or using the pull-down menus, it is likely that you will want to keep a record of your commands so that you can refer to them (and run them again) later. For those familiar with the syntax window in SPSS, the do file editor in Stata is much the same.

If you click on the do file editor icon at the top of the Stata window – ✍ ▾ in version 9 and 🗋 ▾ in version 10 – a do file editor box appears. The do file editor is a simple text editor (similar to Notepad) in which you can type, copy, cut and paste text. In version 10 you may have more than one do file editor open; we suggest you start by only having one open, but note this function for when you are more familiar with the software.

In here you can type your commands and save them, keeping a record of how you have configured your files and manipulated your data. We will focus more on the use of do files later. We recommend using do files as soon as possible but to start out using either the pull-down menus or typing commands into the Command window.

The do file editor in version 10 can have numerous do files open. The open do files are listed as tabs below the toolbar. In this example there are three do files open in the editor: *analysis_10.do*, *org10_1.do*, and *orgbirth_30.do*. The do file currently shown (or at the front) is *analysis_10.do* as the name is in bold, while the other two are dimmed. To bring one of the others to the front simply click on the name.

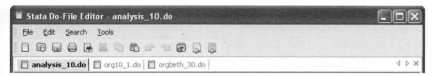

Stata distinguishes between being asked to **do** a command and being asked to **run** a command. Both execute the commands but **do** tells you what command has been used and produces any results as it does them while **run** is silent or not showing the results. This can be a little frustrating when getting to know Stata. To start with we suggest that you use **do** all the time. The **do** icon is the farthest right on the do file editor tool bar ▣ . The one to its left is the **run** icon. If you look closely you can see that the **do** icon has lines on it which indicate output whereas the **run** icon is blank showing that it runs silently.

Under the **Tools** pull-down menu are some other options for **do** and **run**. It is important to understand that if you just click the **do** icon on the toolbar (or choose **Do** from the pull-down menu) then Stata will **do** the whole do file starting from the top. If you only want to **do** a line or two then you can select those lines in the do file then either click the **do** icon on the toolbar (or choose **Do** from the pull-down menu) and Stata will only execute those commands. The last option is to position the cursor in the do file and then use **Do to Bottom** from the pull-down menu. In this case Stata will do all commands from where the cursor is to the end of the do file.

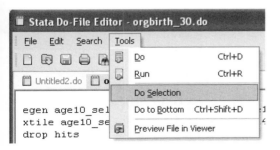

It should be noted here that there are other text editors that people use to save their commands, but for the purposes of this book, we will use the editor provided in Stata.

LOG FILES

Because you can't save the contents of the results screen in Stata (like the output window in SPSS, if you have used that program before), you should quickly get into the habit of using log files. Like the name suggests, log files make a record of your Stata session and include all your commands and results in one document. You will find an icon – ⊗ in version 9 and ▣ in version 10 – on the toolbar which is the button for beginning a log file. We will return to log files in the next chapter, but for now, just remember that these are the types of files we use in Stata to make a record of our session.

Box 1.2: File extensions

There are four file extensions in Stata that you should get to know:

- data files have the extension .dta – this corresponds to .sav files if you might be familiar with in SPSS;
- do files have the extension .do – this is similar to the .sps extension in SPSS for syntax;
- log files have the extension .log or .smcl (Stata Markup and Control Language) – this is most like the output file in SPSS, which has the extension .spo;
- graphs have the extension .gph

WHERE ARE MY DATA?

If you are accustomed to other statistical software, you might be puzzled as to how to view your data. In SPSS, for example, there is a Data Viewer window that is open even while you are using the pull-down menus to select your commands. In Stata, the data is 'behind the scenes', like the log file. If you look on your menu bar, you will see these two icons: ▦ ▨ in version 9 and ▭ ▩ in version 10. The one on the left is the **Data Editor** and the one on the right is the **Data Browser** (with the magnifying glass). You can physically change the data in your data file in the **Data Editor**, but *not* in the **Data Browser**. Only the **Data Editor** or the **Data Browser** may be open at one time (not both). Also, you must close the **Data Editor** and **Data Browser** before Stata will run any commands.

Now that we have an idea of what all the windows are for, it is time to turn to how to really 'get started'. We begin by preparing Stata to work with data and setting up our directories.

ALLOCATING MEMORY TO STATA

When Stata launches, there is a note in the Results window that tells you how much space has been allocated to data. This varies by the flavour of Stata, network and the default settings on your computer/ network. On the particular computer that we use, Stata opens with 1 Mb allocated to memory. This may seem like plenty, but a lot of data sets are much bigger than this and therefore it is necessary to increase the allocation of memory. To use your available memory efficiently we suggest that you set the memory to only slightly larger than the data set to be used. If, for example, we want to change the allocated memory to 50 Mb, we just use the command:

```
set mem 50m
```

You can type whatever amount of memory you require here depending on the size of the data set you are using and the specifications of your computer. If you move on to analysing large survey-type data then you may need to specify 250–500 Mb of memory. If you decide, after some practice, that you typically use 50 Mb (or some other amount) of memory every time you use Stata, you can type

```
set mem 50m, permanently
```

This memory allocation will take effect by default every time you start Stata.

SETTING DIRECTORIES

You can, and should, make sure that all of your files for a particular project are saved to the same directory on your computer. This will make it easier to retrieve any file related to a particular project and save you retyping long file locations every time you want to open or save data.

You can tell Stata to create a directory using the command **mkdir** (make directory) – a new directory is created where you can store all of our data, syntax, and log files. So if you type in the command window:

mkdir c:/projectname

Stata will make a folder in your C drive called projectname. Of course, you would want to change this to where you want your data and do files stored. It might not be on the C drive and you probably would want a more meaningful name for your folder! Alternatively, you can create the folder you want to use first through your software and its file and folder management functions.

You can then use the command **cd** to tell Stata to change directory so that your files are stored there. Type:

cd c:/projectname

In version 10 you can change the working directory using the pull-down menu:

File → Change working directory

Then browse to the location of the directory/folder you wish to use.

Now if you save any files without explicitly defining another directory, your files will be saved in this directory. So if you have a data set open and you want to save it, you can simply just type **save nameofdata** and this file would now appear in your new directory.

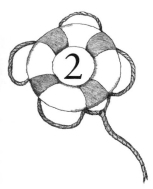

Data in and out of Stata

2

OPENING A STATA DATA FILE

To open an existing Stata data file you can either:

(1) use the **Open** icon on the toolbar and browse to the file location;
(2) use the pull-down menu **File → Open** and browse to the file location; or
(3) type in the Command window or a do file:
    use datafilename.dta,clear

If you use method (1) or (2) when another data set is already open, Stata will warn you if those data have been changed and ask you either to clear the current data without saving the changes or to cancel the opening of the new data set. If you do want to save the changes then cancel and save the open data before opening the new data.

In method (3), the **clear** option tells Stata to clear any existing data before opening the data file specified in the command. Only use the **clear** option when you are absolutely sure you want to clear out any open data in its current state. The **clear** option is not necessary when opening the first data file after launching Stata when no other data are open. Stata will return an error message and stop if the **clear** is omitted and other data are open. If you haven't changed the default colours for fonts, error messages are returned in red, and the error message will say (in red): no; data in memory would be lost.

Version 10 uses **clear** and **clear all** commands in different circumstances, and as you become more familiar with Stata you will be able to use the **clear** options more efficiently.

In (3) you do not have to specify the path to the data file if you have changed directories using the **cd** command to the location of the data file. In some cases it is preferable to read the master data from one location, such as when using a read-only data library, and then store smaller data files for analysis and output results in another location. For this kind of scenario we recommend using the **cd** command to point Stata to the location of the directory you wish to use to store your analysis data files and results, and then when opening the master data specify the whole path. An example of the series of commands where you wish to read master data from a data library but put all other files in a project folder on your local drive would be:

```
cd "C:\projects\project_a"
use "M:\datalibrary\masterdata.dta",clear
```

The first line instructs Stata to use the project_a folder on your C drive as the default directory, so unless otherwise specified all **use** and **save** commands retrieve or place files in that folder. The second line retrieves the master data file from the data library and opens it in Stata.

You will notice that Stata repeats the **cd "C:\projects\ project_a"** command in the Results window in yellow. Unlike messages returned in red, which are error messages, yellow messages are result messages which give you feedback on what you have just done. You will also see that the **cd** and **use** commands are entered in white in the Results window, as this is the default colour for inputs (what you type). When you start producing results in the Results window, you will see that the majority of type here is green, as that is the default results colour.

After you have opened a data file you will see a list of variables in the Variables window. The variable names are listed on the left while the labels are on the right. Sometimes you have to expand the right-hand side of this window to see all the variable labels, particularly if they are quite long. Providing you have your windows set up in a similar way, the screen shot shows you how your screen may look after opening a data file. If your data are blank in the area for variable labels, this means that there were no labels assigned to the variables or that they were lost when you transferred your data into Stata. We show you how to add these later in the book. Also note that the command to open the data is repeated in the Results window and in the Review window. What you will see in the Review window depends on whether you are typing the command into the Command window or using a command in a do file. If it is the former, the command you typed will appear there. If it is the latter, you will see a line in the review window that starts with do but is then followed by a file directory, which is pointing to the location of the do file being used.

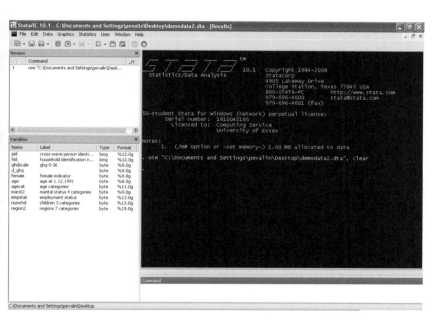

You can see that the data file demodata2.dta has 11 variables. With a small number of variables it is possible to manage the whole file quite easily. However, if you use large data files, such as survey data, and you do not need to open the data with all of the variables then you can modify the **use** command to select which variables you choose. For example, if we only wanted to open the variables *female* and *empstat* from the demodata2.dta file then we would type in the Command window or do file:

```
use female empstat using demodata2.dta, clear
```

For different ways of exploring your data, see Box 2.1.

Keep and drop

There are two commands that allow you to specify the variables you wish to keep in the open data set once you have opened the

Box 2.1: Inspecting your data

If you type **codebook** into the Command window, you will be presented with information about variables' names, labels, and values. The default setting is to provide this information about all of the variables in your data set. If you wish to see the information from only a few then specify the variables after the command. For example:

```
. codebook sex age

--------------------------------------------------------
sex
--------------------------------------------------------

            type:  numeric (byte)
           label:  asex

           range:  [1,2]                units:  1
   unique values:  2              missing .:  0/10264

      tabulation:  Freq.   Numeric Label
                   4833           1 male
                   5431           2 female

--------------------------------------------------------
age
--------------------------------------------------------

            type:  numeric (byte)
           label:  aage12, but 81 nonmissing
                   values are not labeled

           range:  [16,97]              units:  1
   unique values:  81             missing .:  0/10264

        examples:  27
                   37
                   47
                   63
```

In version 10 the **codebook** command has an option – **compact** or **c** – that produces a briefer description of the variables. The same variables – *sex* and *age* – are shown in compact form below.

```
. codebook sex age,c

Variable    Obs   Unique      Mean   Min Max   Label
-------------------------------------------------------------
sex        10264        2  1.529131     1    2   sex
age        10264       81  44.41553    15   96   age at date
                                                 of interview
-------------------------------------------------------------
```

The command **inspect** is also useful for checking data accuracy. Again the default is to provide all variables, so specify those for which you require the information. For example:

```
. inspect sex age

sex: sex                            Number of Observations
--------                            --------------------------

                              Total  Integers  Nonintegers
|    #          Negative         -         -           -
| #  #          Zero             -         -           -
| #  #          Positive     10264     10264           -
| #  #                        -----     -----       -----
| #  #          Total        10264     10264           -
| #  #          Missing         -
+-----------                  -----
1          2                  10264
   (2 unique values)

   sex is labeled and all values are documented
   in the label.

age: age                            Number of Observations
--------                            --------------------------

                              Total  Integers  Nonintegers
| #             Negative         -         -           -
| #  #          Zero             -         -           -
| #  #          Positive     10264     10264           -
| #  #  #                     -----     -----       -----
| #  #  #  #    Total        10264     10264           -
| #  #  #  # .  Missing         -
+-----------                  -----
16         97                 10264
   (81 unique values)

   age is labeled but 10264 values are NOT
   documented in the label.
```

full data. The command **keep** is followed by a list of variables you wish to keep in the open data. For example:

keep sex age educ

The command **drop** is also followed by a list of variables but this time those that you wish to remove from the open data. For example:

drop pid hid region-ghq

If there is a group of variables you wish to either **keep** or **drop** then you can just put the first and last variable as listed in the Variables window with a dash between and Stata will read this as including all variables between the two named in the order they are in the variables window. This notation can be used in other commands as well.

OPENING OTHER TYPES OF DATA FILES

There are a number of commands to help you import data in other formats but here we concentrate on probably the two most common formats: Excel spreadsheets and SPSS data files. See Box 2.2 for a software package which converts many different forms of data.

> **Box 2.2: Stat/Transfer**
>
> Stat/Transfer is a software package that converts data files from one format to another. There are too many formats to list here but all commonly used spreadsheets (Excel, Access, dBase etc.) and statistical packages (Stata, SPSS, SAS, Epi Info, etc.) are covered. See www.stattransfer.com and www.stata.com/products/transfer.html.

Excel spreadsheets

If you have data in an Excel spreadsheet and want to transfer it into Stata, from where you can save it as a Stata data file (.dta), you will have to go through a few intermediate steps. You can then either use the pull-down menus or use the **insheet** command in the Command window or a do file. These instructions assume you have your data organized in Excel with the variable names in the first row and then one case or respondent's data per row.

With your data open in Excel you need to save it as a text (tab delimited) file with a .txt extension. You can do this by using **File → Save As** and then selecting the type of file to save.

If you choose to use the pull-down menus in Stata to open the data then use

File → Import → ASCII data created by spreadsheet

and then click **Browse** to go to the location of the .txt file. There are a few options available to you at this stage but if your data are organized as above then you do not need to change any of the default settings. When you browse to find the .txt file, you need to make sure that the you can see **Files of type: All(*.*)** set in the lower panel of the **Open** dialogue box.

Click on **OK** and the data should open with your list of variables in the Variables window. You can visually check your data by clicking the **Data Browser** button (see Chapter 1) on the toolbar and inspect the spreadsheet.

If you wish to use the Command window or put commands in a do file use:

```
insheet datafile.txt, clear
```

This assumes the .txt file is in the default Stata directory or you can enter the path to the file.

To save your data in Stata format (.dta) see the **Saving data** section below.

SPSS data files

Until recently SPSS data files had to be converted manually, in a similar way to Excel spreadsheets, but now there is the command **usespss** which allows you to open an SPSS for windows (.sav) datafile directly in Stata. Type:

```
findit usespss
```

Then follow the instructions to install the command.

The **usespss** command works in a similar way to the usual Stata commands for opening existing files (see above):

```
usespss using "pathandfilename", clear
```

After opening the data it can be saved in Stata format (.dta). See the **Saving data** section below.

If you are using version 9.0 then you will need to obtain the free update to version 9.2 for the command to work. Type **update query** in the Command window and follow the instructions.

The latest versions of SPSS can save data in Stata format (.dta).

ENTERING YOUR OWN DATA INTO STATA

It may be the case that you have raw data that you want to enter directly into Stata. As mentioned in Chapter 1, look for the following two icons: 🖽 🗹 or 🗔 🗔 on the menu bar. The one on the left is the **Data Editor** and the one on the right is the **Data Browser**. The **Data Editor** is the one you will want to open in order to enter your own data. Once you launch the **Data Editor**, you can proceed to add your own data. The variables go in columns, with each row representing a single observation. Here, you can enter text and numbers, depending on the nature of your variables. To save the inputted data, click **Preserve** in the top left-hand corner. You will see that new variables are listed for you in the variables window. You will need to label the variables and their categories (if applicable) using commands that are covered in Chapter 3.

SAVING DATA

To save your data at any time under a new file name you can either:

(1)   use the pull-down menu **File** → **Save As** and browse to the location you wish to save the file and enter its new name; or
(2)   type in the Stata Command window or do file if you wish to save the data in the default directory or the one you have previously specified with the **cd** command:
```
save newdata.dta
```

If you wish to overwrite an existing data file with a modified version then add the option **replace**:

```
save newdata.dta, replace
```

When you are using a do file (and remember that we strongly recommend you progress to using them as soon as possible) it is preferable to use the **replace** option all the time. This is because if the option is not used and a data file with that name already exists then the **save** command will cause an error (returned in red and indicating that the file already exists) and the do file commands will stop at that point. If the option is used the first time a data file with that name is saved, Stata will report a (green) message that states that the file you indicated could not be found to be replaced. This isn't a problem – Stata is just telling you that it couldn't literally replace a file because one by that particular name wasn't already in existence, but it will save it anyway and continue with the next command in the do file. But the next time you run the file and make changes to the original data file, you will see that Stata will overwrite previous versions with the **replace** option. See Box 2.3 for a discussion of the importance of careful data file management.

Box 2.3: Overwriting your data

If you regularly use master data drawn from a read-only data library then you need only be concerned with whether to or when to overwrite your data for analysis files. This is because the system will not allow you to overwrite the master data. If you have your own data master files on your local drive you run the risk of accidentally overwriting those files, especially when you are in the early stages of getting to know a new software package.

After going to all the trouble of collecting, coding and entering your own data you need to guard against ruining that work. We recommend that you keep a master copy in a place detached from your local drive (CD-ROM, USB drive, or a networked remote drive) and, to be doubly sure, designate the copy of the master data that you are using on your local drive as read-only.

LOG FILES

We mentioned log files briefly in the previous chapter. A log file keeps a record of your commands and results during a Stata session. At first you may wonder why this is necessary as the results are shown immediately in the Results window on your screen. The Results window has a limited capacity, and while you might initially find that this is sufficient for your use (or you may increase the buffer size to be much greater), you will quickly need the capacity to permanently record your sessions as your data manipulation and analysis becomes more complex.

You need to explicitly tell Stata when to open a log file and to close it. This may seem odd to those familiar with SPSS, where an output window automatically opens when the first command is executed, but we believe it does give a greater degree of flexibility for complex series of analyses. In Stata you can open a log file at any time, close it, open it again to add further results, or open a new log file altogether. We find this particularly useful when we want to separate results from data manipulation or when preparing tables for a report where it is possible to produce a log file for the analysis for each table rather than one larger log file. Of course, you may prefer one large log file with clear annotations separating the different stages of the analysis, and Stata has the flexibility to manage either.

Log files come in two formats; both have their advantages and disadvantages. You specify the format you want by the extension to the log file name – this can be either **.log** or **.scml** – when you tell Stata to open a log file.

If you chose to use the log file with **.smcl** format (this is the default, so if you do not specify a file extension then you will get this format) then you can view this file by using the **View** option from the **File** pull-down menu in Stata and browsing to the log file. The **.smcl** log files have the same properties as the results that are displayed in the Results window. This file format also has the advantage that is can be copied and pasted easily into Excel and Word, which is a topic that we will return to in later in this chapter.

Log files with a **.log** extension are text files that can be viewed in any word processor. The downside is that it is not as easy to copy and paste tables to Excel, and to view them correctly you need to ensure that the font is one with equal spaces for each character such as **Courier**. To view your log file in Word, remember to select **Display all file types** when you are searching for your file, as its file extension is not .doc.

If you wish to only record what you type into the Command window, then you can open, close, turn on and off a command log file using **cmdlog** instead of **log**. You can have command logs open at the same time as normal log files if you wish.

Starting a log file

The command **log using** starts a log file, and you tell Stata the name you wish to call it (e.g. analysis) and which format you want. Assuming you wish to save the log file in the directory you have previously specified using the **cd** command, you would use:

```
log using analysis.log,replace
```

or

```
log using analysis.scml,replace
```

The **replace** option is used to overwrite the original file with a modified version. In a similar way to using the **replace** option with the **save** command, if **replace** is not specified and a file by that name exists, Stata will show an error and stop the do file. If **replace** is used and there is no file by that name Stata will show a warning the first time the file is created but then carry on with the next command in the do file.

   If you are using the pull-down menus or the Command window and still want to keep a log file of your commands and results then you can use the log file icon on the toolbar – 🗶 in version 9 and 📄 in version 10 – to open, suspend and close a log file.

   When you open a log file, Stata automatically records the location of the log file, the type of log file and the time and date it was opened at the beginning of the file. For example:

```
. log using "C:\Documents and
               Settings\project_a\analysis.log"
       log:  C:\Documents and
               Settings\project_a\analysis.log
  log type:  text
 opened on:  19 Oct 2007, 11:32:41
```

Closing a log file

When you close a log file it is saved to the location specified when you opened it with the **log using** command. To close the log file, simply type:

```
log close
```

and Stata records the location of the log file, the type of log file and the time and date the log file was closed at the end of the file. For example:

```
. log close
       log:  C:\Documents and
                Settings\project_a\analysis.log
  log type:  text
 closed on:  19 Oct 2007, 11:53:23
```

The **log close** command shuts the log file completely, and if you want to reopen it to add more information then you need to type **log using** with **append** (as below).

However, if you want to just turn off the log temporarily then you can use **log off** and then **log on** to turn it back on later in your analysis or in your do file. After the **log off** command is used Stata records when the log was paused:

```
. log off
      log:  C:\Documents and Settings\
              project_a\analysis.log
  log type:  text
 paused on:  19 Oct 2007, 12:03:35
```

After the **log on** command Stata records when the log was resumed:

```
. log on
      log:  C:\Documents and Settings\
              project_a\analysis.log
  log type:  text
resumed on:  19 Oct 2007, 12:13:51
```

Adding to your log file

If you want to reopen an existing log file and add further results to it, rather than overwrite it as with the **replace** subcommand, you open the log file in the usual way but use an **append** option:

log using analysis.log,append

and Stata records the location, type and time and date the new results were added to the log file in the same way as when the log file was first opened.

COPYING RESULTS TO EXCEL AND WORD

Tables and other forms of analysis results can be copied from the Results window straight into Excel and Word to create tables in your documents and spreadsheets. In this example, two variables, marital status (*mastat*) and gender (*sex*) from our example data are crosstabulated using the **tabulate** command (see Chapter 6 for a further discussion of this command):

```
. tabulate mastat sex

                              sex
  marital status       male      female  |      Total
         married      2,947       3,062  |      6,009
living as couple        334         340  |        674
         widowed        169         697  |        866
        divorced        150         284  |        434
       separated         59         130  |        189
   never married      1,174         918  |      2,092
           Total      4,833       5,431  |     10,264
```

Use the cursor and mouse to highlight the table:

```
. tabulate mastat sex

                              sex
  marital status       male      female        Total
         married      2,947       3,062        6,009
living as couple        334         340          674
         widowed        169         697          866
        divorced        150         284          434
       separated         59         130          189
   never married      1,174         918        2,092
           Total      4,833       5,431       10,264
```

Either right-click and choose **Copy table** or use the **Edit** pull down menu to do the same.

In Excel, choose one cell and then right-click and choose **Paste** or use the **Edit** pull-down menu to do the same. The data will be automatically entered in their own cells in the Excel spreadsheet:

	A	B	C	D
1				
2		sex		
3	marital status	male	female	Total
4				
5	married	2,947	3,062	6,009
6	living as couple	334	340	674
7	widowed	169	697	866
8	divorced	150	284	434
9	separated	59	130	189
10	never married	1,174	918	2,092
11				
12	Total	4,833	5,431	10,264
13				

In Word, **Paste** the data into the document. It will appear spaced by tabs, and to convert it to a table you need to select the rows and go to **Table** → **Convert** → **Text to table**. The default settings will be OK to change the pasted data into a table in Word.

FILE MANAGEMENT

In Figure 2.1 we illustrate the main routes for your Stata commands (whether these are generated by a pull-down menu, Command window or do file), data and results when you are working with master data in a read-only library. This could easily be adapted in the case where your master data are held in a read-only folder on your local drive (see our recommendations in Box 2.3).

There are probably as many ways of organizing analysis files as there are researchers, but we would like to suggest two main ways as a starting point for your own file management system. We would like to stress the importance of adopting a systematic approach to file management and archiving whatever system you finally decide to use. This can pay dividends, as one of us (DP) found out (see Box 2.4).

The first approach is to group files by project. In this way all data files, do files and log files are in the same project folder. This allows you to specify the project folder in the **cd** command knowing that all files for that project are there to access, overwrite or save. This system works well provided the number of files does not become unwieldy. A way of dealing with large numbers of files is to adopt a system of prefixing your file names in order to group types of files. As the default way of showing files in a folder using Windows is alphabetical on the file name, if you use *do_*, *data_*, and *log_* to start names for do files, data files and log files respectively, then they will be shown in those groups. We also recommend that you try to be systematic in the naming of files,

Figure 2.1

Information flow

schematic

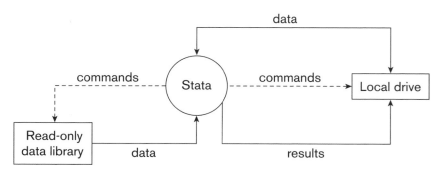

Box 2.4: The importance of good file management

In 2003 I (DP) analysed data from an American panel study (the National Longitudinal Study of Adolescent Health[1] – AddHealth) for a paper which was eventually published in 2005.[2] In the summer of 2006 I was contacted by a researcher who was doing a meta-review of studies that had looked at cannabis use and depression.[3] As this was one of the aspects of our paper, the researcher had questions about the measures and methods we had used, as well as asking for some additional results that were not published, such as bivariate odds ratios where we had only published multivariate results.

When I think back to when I started data analysis and my rather haphazard file management, such a request then would have caused me hours of work trawling back through badly named and annotated files to find the particular statistics needed for this meta review. But this time, because I had adopted a file management system and had copiously annotated my do files, I was able to find the information and provide the unpublished results in a matter of minutes.

Most of the time the annotations on do files and their systematic use and storage will not be called on as mine were, but they are an investment which you may well be required to cash in sometime in the future. The time between submission to a journal and receiving reviews that may ask for additional analysis can be quite substantial, and you may have gone on to other projects in that time. Good annotations will allow you to get back into the analysis much faster than trying to work through each command line to try and remember what you had done all those many months ago.

[1] Udry, J.R. (2003) The National Longitudinal Study of Adolescent Health (Add Health), Waves I & II, 1994–1996; Wave III, 2001–2002 [machine-readable data file and documentation]. Chapel Hill, NC: Carolina Population Center, University of North Carolina at Chapel Hill.
[2] Wade, T.J. and Pevalin, D.J. (2005) Adolescent delinquency and health. *Canadian Journal of Criminology and Criminal Justice*, 47: 619–654.
[3] Moore, T.H.M., Zammit, S., Lingford-Hughes, A. et al. (2007) Cannabis use and risk of psychotic or affective mental health outcomes: a systematic review. *Lancet*, 370 (9584): 319–328.

especially do files and log files, so that it is obvious what stage of the project they relate to. For example, we might have one do file for extracting data from master files, one do file for manipulating those data to construct variables for analysis, and then three do files for analysis. In this case we would name the do files as follows:

do_extraction.do
do_construction.do
do_analysis_1.do
do_analysis_2.do
do_analysis_3.do

If you do not like the prefixing of the file names then you can click on the **Type** column top button in Windows, when in **List** or **Detail** view, and the files in that folder will be grouped by their extensions.

The second approach which we use for larger projects is to set up three subfolders in the project folder: one for do files, one for data, and one for log files. This way does not allow you to easily use the **cd** command to specify a single folder, but long paths can easily be copied and pasted in the do file editor. When using this system it is important to be able to identify which log files come from which do files. We use numbers to link them so that *analysis_1.do* produces *results_1.log*, and if there is more than one log file from a single do file we would use letters to distinguish them such as *results_1a.log*, *results_1b.log*.

USING THESE COMMANDS IN A DO FILE

Below we provide a starting template for a standard beginning and end of a do file. This starting template is for a single do file producing a single log file. Do files can be much more complex than this basic example, and we would expect you to develop and tailor your do files as you gain more experience with Stata. For example, you may have a number of log files open at the same time, in different formats, and then pause, resume and close each of them at separate times. In this case the **name(tempname)** option is very useful, but for now remembering that this is possible is enough to be going on with.

Explanations of the commands are annotated in the do file in the ways that can be actually used to annotate and note do files so they are more meaningful. You can add comments in do files which give an explanation of the commands you have written. These can be handy when you go back to a do file months later and can't remember why you did certain things. Indeed, you probably will not appreciate the importance of commenting until you have experienced this type of frustration. It is certainly better to have more comments than not enough! Any line that begins with an asterisk will be ignored by Stata as a command. If your comment extends for numerous lines, you will have to make sure that every line begins with *, or you can use a different technique for extensive commenting, writing /* at the beginning of the comment and */ at the end. Anything between these signposts is ignored. It is important, if you decide to use this latter method for extensive commenting, that you remember to put in your end of comment signifier */ or everything after the opening /* will be regarded as a comment – possibly the rest of your do file! Both types of commenting techniques are shown below. For additional commenting techniques, see **help comment**.

```
set mem 10m
version 10.1           /* not required but a good
                       habit to get into in
                       case you have any version-
                       specific commands */
capture log close     /* closes any log files
                       still open */
set more off          /* turns off the need to hit
                       space bar when the Results
                       window is full */
cd M:\projects\project_a\analysis

log using analysis_1.scml,replace
* the .scml is not formally required as it is
* the default format

use id sex age mastat educ using ///
   "K:\datalibrary\data_file",clear

* manipulation and analysis commands here

save analysis_file.dta,replace
* the .dta is not formally required
log close
```

Note that this is the first time we have used the /// notation to indicate that a command line goes over to the next line. This is only
used in do files and not the Command window – see interacting
with Stata in Chapter 1.

Another way of organising your do file would be to only open
the log file when you have analysis results you wish to keep and
exclude the data manipulation. In this case your do file might be
structured as follows:

```
set mem 10m
version 10.1
capture log close
set more off
cd M:\projects\project_a\analysis

use id sex age mastat educ using ///
    "K:\datalibrary\data_file", clear

*first set of manipulation commands here

log using analysis_1.scml, replace

*first set of analysis commands here

log off

*second set of manipulation commands here

log on

*second set of analysis commands here and
*be sure to close log

log close

save analysis_file.dta, replace
```

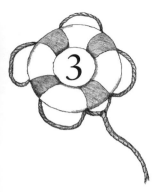

3 Manipulating variables

MANIPULATING VARIABLES – WHY?

Often, when you are working with data, you need to make changes to your variables. This may be for a number of reasons. For example, you may have an income variable that is measured in pounds, but you would prefer to have income grouped into a number of categories, or even percentiles, instead. You may be examining educational qualifications, but you are only really interested in studying whether people went to university or not, and therefore you would collapse a variable into two categories (i.e. went to university, didn't go to university). You may have a very detailed ethnicity or race variable that was collected as an open-ended question – that is, the survey respondents could write in whatever they pleased. Clearly a categorical variable with hundreds of possible responses would be very nearly impossible to work with and therefore you may want to collapse these into more manageable categories. There are many reasons you would want to change the way your variables are presented. One special instance is the case of missing values.

MISSING VALUES

When people answer surveys, they don't always answer all the questions, either because they would rather not or because not all the questions may be relevant to them. Survey researchers use a variety of techniques to capture the instances where a respondent may refuse to answer a question or that question isn't appropriate for the particular respondent. Often these values are recorded in the data spreadsheet as negative numbers, such as −1 for 'refused' or −9 for 'inapplicable'. Sometimes, they are stored as high numbers, such as 99 or 999. There is no rule about this – it depends on the conventions of the particular researcher or research institute who collected the data.

You can recode the missing values to one or more of the 27 values Stata recognizes as meaning 'missing'. These 27 are a dot (.) and a dot followed by a letter (.a to .z). Stata actually uses the dot to recode the value to an extremely high number, which is why you have to be careful when using the greater than symbol (>) if the variable has missing values.

In our example data the data collectors decided to use negative numbers (i.e. −7, −8) to indicate non-response for a variety of reasons. The table below shows the output of the variable *educ* using the **tabulate** command (see Chapter 5):

```
. tabulate educ
```

highest educational qualification	Freq.	Percent	Cum.
missing	19	0.19	0.19
proxy respondent	352	3.43	3.61
higher degree	122	1.19	4.80
first degree	598	5.83	10.63
teaching qf	225	2.19	12.82
other higher qf	1,207	11.76	24.58
nursing qf	215	2.09	26.68
gce a levels	985	9.60	36.27
gce o levels or equiv	2,086	20.32	56.60
commercial qf, no o levels	349	3.40	60.00
cse grade 2-5, scot grade 4-5	411	4.00	64.00
apprenticeship	262	2.55	66.55
other qf	84	0.82	67.37
no qf	3,349	32.63	100.00
Total	10,264	100.00	

As you can see from the frequency table there are 19 cases with 'missing' values and 352 cases where this question was asked of a 'proxy respondent'. A proxy respondent is someone in the household who answers questions on the respondent's behalf if he or she is not able to participate. If we tabulate again, with the option **nol** (nolabel) asking for the values rather than the labels of the categories, we get:

```
. tabulate educ,nol

      highest |
   educational |
 qualification |      Freq.     Percent        Cum.
---------------+---------------------------------
           -9 |         19        0.19        0.19
           -7 |        352        3.43        3.61
            1 |        122        1.19        4.80
            2 |        598        5.83       10.63
            3 |        225        2.19       12.82
            4 |      1,207       11.76       24.58
            5 |        215        2.09       26.68
            6 |        985        9.60       36.27
            7 |      2,086       20.32       56.60
            8 |        349        3.40       60.00
            9 |        411        4.00       64.00
           10 |        262        2.55       66.55
           11 |         84        0.82       67.37
           12 |      3,349       32.63      100.00
---------------+---------------------------------
        Total |     10,264      100.00
```

We see that −9 is the value given to 'missing' cases and −7 to 'proxy respondent' cases. For this variable we would choose to recode both −9 and −7 to be missing values.

There are a number of ways to specify missing values. The first uses the **recode** command, where we recode both the negative numbers to a dot.

recode educ -9=. -7=.

or

recode educ -9/-7=.

The forward slash **/** is Stata notation for a range of values – in the above example, values −9 through −7. Remember to put the lowest value first. There are no cases with a value of −8, but that doesn't matter.

If you wanted to keep the reasons for the missing values separate then you could use the dot followed by a letter values such as

```
recode educ −9=.a −7=.b
```

Also, you can recode more than one variable at a time if the variables in your list have the same values to change. For example, if our variables education (*educ*) and housing tenure (*tenure*) had the same range of missing values to recode, we could use

```
recode educ tenure (−9/−1=.)
```

or

```
recode educ tenure (−9=.a) (−7=.b)
```

Where there is more than one variable in the list, the recode values must be in parentheses. The **recode** command is also used to manipulate the non-missing values of variables, and this is covered in the next section.

You must be sure that the 'missing' values do not have a *meaningful value*. That is, in our example data, when the negative values you may think to recode to missing values can represent a real value, such as zero, for a variable. To illustrate this we shall look at the variables *ncigs*, which measures how many cigarettes a respondent smoked per day.

First, let us get some descriptive information on the variable.

```
. ta ncigs
```

number of cigarettes smoked	Freq.	Percent	Cum.
missing or wild	20	0.19	0.19
inapplicable	6,949	67.70	67.90
proxy respondent	352	3.43	71.33
refused	1	0.01	71.34
don't know	1	0.01	71.35
less than 1 per day	41	0.40	71.75
1	39	0.38	72.13
2	55	0.54	72.66
3	50	0.49	73.15
4	31	0.30	73.45
5	162	1.58	75.03

```
             6 |        59        0.57       75.60
             7 |        53        0.52       76.12
             8 |        62        0.60       76.72
             9 |        14        0.14       76.86
            10 |       501        4.88       81.74

           etc
            60 |         9        0.09       99.99
            80 |         1        0.01      100.00
---------------+----------------------------------
         Total |    10,264      100.00
```

We can see that several respondents smoked less than one per day.
We can find out the variable values as well.

```
. ta ncigs,nol

    number of |
   cigarettes |
       smoked |     Freq.     Percent       Cum.
--------------+----------------------------------
           -9 |        20        0.19        0.19
           -8 |     6,949       67.70       67.90
           -7 |       352        3.43       71.33
           -2 |         1        0.01       71.34
           -1 |         1        0.01       71.35
            0 |        41        0.40       71.75
            1 |        39        0.38       72.13
            2 |        55        0.54       72.66
            3 |        50        0.49       73.15
            4 |        31        0.30       73.45
            5 |       162        1.58       75.03
            6 |        59        0.57       75.60
            7 |        53        0.52       76.12
            8 |        62        0.60       76.72
            9 |        14        0.14       76.86
           10 |       501        4.88       81.74

          etc
           60 |         9        0.09       99.99
           80 |         1        0.01      100.00
--------------+----------------------------------
        Total |    10,264      100.00
```

All respondents were asked the question 'Do you smoke?'. If they answered 'Yes', then they were asked the second question, 'How many cigarettes do you smoke a day?'. If they answered 'No' to the first question then they were not asked the second question. This can be seen by the number of respondents with a value of −8 in the variable *ncigs*. This number should correspond to the number of respondents who answered 'No' to the first question. As well, there is a value of 0, which is labelled as less than 1 per day. But these are occasional smokers, so are they really zeros?

If you wanted a variable that indicated the number of cigarettes smoked per day then you could recode the negative values of *ncigs* in this way:

```
recode ncigs 0=1 −9=. −8=0 −7=. −2=. −1=.
```

Or, if you wanted to keep the reasons for missing values separate:

```
recode ncigs 0=1 −9=.a −8=0 −7=.b −2=.c −1=.d
```

In the second way we have kept **−9=.a** and **−7=.b** as they are for the *educ* variable, as in our data −9 and −7 denote the same reason for missing values in all of the variables. Both of these recodes will produce the frequency table of the *ncigs* variable below. The differences in coding the missing values are only shown when the **missing** option is used in the **tabulate** command which we cover in Chapter 5.

```
. ta ncigs,nol
```

number of cigarettes smoked	Freq.	Percent	Cum.
0	6,949	70.26	70.26
1	80	0.81	71.07
2	55	0.56	71.63
3	50	0.51	72.13
4	31	0.31	72.45
5	162	1.64	74.08
6	59	0.60	74.68
7	53	0.54	75.22
8	62	0.63	75.84

```
 9 |          14        0.14        75.99
10 |         501        5.07        81.05

etc
60 |           9        0.09        99.99
80 |           1        0.01       100.00
-----------+----------------------------
Total |   9,890      100.00
```

There is a useful command that will convert all the negative values to missing values in one step. But before you use this global recode, you must make sure that all the values that you are going to specify are *indeed logically deemed to be system missing* and you want to recode all of the missing values to a dot (.) only rather than keep the reasons for missing values separate. The command is **mvdecode** (missing value decode). The subcommand is **_all** (for all variables) and the further option **mv** specifies which value(s) to treat as missing.

```
mvdecode _all,mv(−9/−1)
```

The shortened range for the missing values (−9/−1) does not work on some Stata configurations. If this is the case with your set-up, then you can enter the missing values one at a time:

```
mvdecode _all,mv(−9)
mvdecode _all,mv(−8)
```
etc.

Also, the **mvdecode** command can be used with single variables or lists of variables and does not have to be used with **_all**:

```
mvdecode mastat,mv(−9/−1)
mvdecode tenure-fimn,mv(−9/−7)
```

The use of negative numbers to indicate values likely to be changed to missing is good practice. It has its limitations, as we have shown above. Another time when negative numbers are not appropriate is when you have standardized scores, as these variables have negative numbers as legitimate values. As we mentioned previously, some data sets use high numbers such as 99 or 999 to indicate non-response (no answer). Additional care is needed when recoding these to missing and especially using the global recode command **mvdecode**. For example, your data may have a variable for age that uses 999 as the indicator for non-response as well as a variable for five categories of marital status that uses 9 as the value for non-response. If you simply used the global **mvdecode _all** command for the range 9/999 then all respondents aged 9 and over would be given a missing value in the age variable. Whatever system is used to indicate non-response, you need to exercise care when declaring values to be missing.

It is very important to note that there is no way to undo the **mvdecode** command. You are well advised to be absolutely sure you want to run this command. And you should *never* overwrite your original data sets – always work with copies.

As you may have gathered by now – there are usually half a dozen different ways to do what you want to do in Stata. As you become more familiar with its possibilities you will find the way that suits you best. In the numerous courses that we have taught on Stata, not one has passed without a student showing us something that we didn't know!

CREATING NEW VARIABLES OUT OF EXISTING VARIABLES

You may want to make new variables out of one or more existing variables. For example, you might want a variable that denotes women who are self-employed. To make this variable, you would need information from two variables that already existed in your data set: gender (*sex*) and job status (*jbstat*).

When you are creating variables, you often need to use mathematical expressions. The following are recognized by Stata:

+   addition
-    subtraction
*   multiplication
/   division
^   raise to the power

Parentheses are used to control the order in which calculations are done. Parentheses may be nested within other parentheses, many layers deep.

Before moving on to more advanced variable manipulation, it is necessary to understand the logical operators used in Stata.

~	not	>	greater than
==	equal (two equals signs)	>=	greater than or equal to
!=	not equal	<	less than
&	and	<=	less than or equal to
|	or		

Stata also recognizes a myriad of mathematical functions. The ones you probably use most are:

sqrt(x)	square root	log(x) or ln(x)	natural logarithm
exp(x)	exponent (*e* to power)	int(x)	integer

Type **help functions** for the full range of functions supported by Stata.

> **Box 3.1: Shortening commands**
>
> The shortening of commands can be used on almost all commands. The manuals or the **help** command will tell you what is the shortest accepted form of the command as shown by the underlined part of the word. For example, **tabulate** can be shortened to **ta**. Some commands cannot be shortened.
>
> However, with **help**, you must spell the name of the command completely, so **help tabulate** will yield you results, while **help tab** will produce a message stating that the command could not be found. Help brings up the online help system for the command. Think of it as the computer version of the Stata manuals, as it often contains the same information! As well, the **search** command looks for the term you indicate in help files, Stata Technical Bulletins, and Stata FAQ if your Stata is web active.

Probably the most common command used to create new variables from pre-existing variables is **generate**. The command **generate** can be shortened to **gen, ge** or even **g**. To use the **generate** command, you type **generate** followed by the name of the new variable and then the set of conditions that equal the value of the new variable. For example, if we wanted to create a variable that measured yearly income, we could multiply our monthly income variable (*fimn*) by 12:

```
gen yearlyincome=fimn*12
```

Likewise, we could generate a variable that roughly equated to weekly income by dividing monthly income by, say, 4.2:

```
ge weeklyincome=fimn/4.2
```

We can use the **recode** command to make a new variable out of an existing variable. Suppose we wanted to make a simplified variable where the only categories were 'partnered', 'never married', and 'previously married' from the original marital status variable (*mastat*). 'Partnered' would include married and cohabiting couples, while 'previously married' would include all divorced, separated, and widowed people. We could do this by:

```
recode mastat 1/2=1 3/5=2 6=3
```

But this would mean that we lose the original variable categories, so we advise that you create new variables when recoding. Let's call our new variable *mastat2*, so now the command will be:

```
recode mastat 1/2=1 3/5=2 6=3,gen(mastat2)
```

The **gen** option to the **recode** command creates a new variable with the recoded categories, so you will keep the original variable and its categories as well.

```
. ta mastat2

mastat2 |     Freq.    Percent       Cum.
--------+-----------------------------------
      1 |     6,683      65.11      65.11
      2 |     1,489      14.51      79.62
      3 |     2,092      20.38     100.00
--------+-----------------------------------
  Total |    10,264     100.00
```

You should always check the variables you create. One way is to crosstabulate them, provided the number of categories is manageable:

```
. ta mastat mastat2
```

marital status	mastat2 1	2	3	Total
married	6,009	0	0	6,009
living as couple	674	0	0	674
widowed	0	866	0	866
divorced	0	434	0	434
separated	0	189	0	189
never married	0	0	2,081	2,081
Total	6,683	1,489	2,081	10,253

Generating a new variable with information from one existing variable is the simplest type of variable creation. Returning to our example of a variable that indicates women who are self-employed, we could do this in a number of different ways; we first use step-by-step approaches so you can see how the different commands work, and then we use a single command to demonstrate Stata's use of logic in constructing new variables. The self-employed have the value 1 in the *jbstat* variable (10 categories) and the missing values have been recoded to a dot (.), while women have the value 2 in the *sex* variable and there are no missing values on the *sex* variable.

The step-by-step way is to generate a new variable (*fem1*) and set all values to missing (.), and then to **replace** the values as they meet specific conditions. The command **replace** allows you to change the contents of a variable, so to speak.

```
gen fem1=.
replace fem1=1 if jbstat==1 & sex==2

replace fem1=0 if jbstat>=2 & jbstat<=12
replace fem1=0 if sex==1 & jbstat==1
```

This will create a value of 1 for all women who are self-employed. You are then left to decide what to do with the rest of the values. A variable must take more than one value to vary. Often, a researcher will use dummy variables to denote 1 for the category of interest and 0 for cases that do not meet this condition, so we replace the new variable with zeros where the cases are women who are not self-employed and all men. The third line replaces those who have an employment status but are not self employed with a 0. The fourth line replaces men who are self-employed with a 0. The step-by-step way of creating this new variable is cumbersome, but it does help to understand what is actually happening in your data with each command. However, we hope that you are able to move quickly on to use more efficient commands.

We can first reduce the four commands to three:

```
gen fem2=1 if jbstat==1 & sex==2
replace fem2=0 if jbstat>=2 & jbstat<=12
replace fem2=0 if sex==1 & jbstat==1
```

In the first command line the **generate** (**gen**) command creates a new variable *fem2* with cases equal to 1 for women who are self-employed, and then the rest of the cases are automatically set as missing (.). The last two command lines are the same as in the first way, replacing all cases that are not self-employed or are self-employed men with a zero. Note here that we do not use **jbstat!=1** (*jbstat* not equal to one) as this would code the cases who are missing on *jbstat* to zero.

We can now reduce the three commands to two:

```
gen fem3=1 if jbstat==1 & sex==2
replace fem3=0 if ((jbstat>=2&jbstat<=10)| ///
    sex==1) & !missing(jbstat)
```

In this way the last two lines are combined to replace cases who are not self-employed or are men as zeros. It is necessary to include the last element of the command line – **& !missing(jbstat)** – in order not to include men who have missing values on the *jbstat* variable in the zeros. This element means 'not missing values on the *jbstat* variable'.

The most efficient way to create this new variable is to use Stata's logic for constructing new variables which then means it can be done in one command line:

```
gen fem4=jbstat==1 & sex==2 if ///
    !missing(jbstat,sex)
```

In this form of the **gen** command, cases who are self-employed (**jbstat==1**) and women (**sex==2**) are automatically given the value 1 while all other cases are given zeros except for those who are missing on either *jbstat* or *sex* – **if !missing (jbstat,sex)** – in which case they are given a missing value (.). Note the use of the **if** in this way rather than the **&** in the last line of making the *fem3* variable. Including the variable **sex** in the parentheses after **!missing** is not strictly necessary as we know in our data that there are no missing values on that variable.

A check on the summary statistics (see Chapter 5) of the new variables shows that they are identical:

```
. su fem*
Variable |     Obs        Mean    Std. Dev.   Min   Max
---------+--------------------------------------------
    fem1 |    9912   .0204802    .1416433      0     1
    fem2 |    9912   .0204802    .1416433      0     1
    fem3 |    9912   .0204802    .1416433      0     1
    fem4 |    9912   .0204802    .1416433      0     1
```

DUMMY VARIABLES

One very common reason to manipulate pre-existing variables is to create dummy variables, or dichotomous variables, with the values of 0 and 1. Dummy variables are a special case of nominal variables. Remember, nominal variables are those which measure qualitative characteristics such as sex, religion, or marital status. There are two reasons why we use dummy variables, and they are based upon what you should already know about nominal variables:

- The only measure of central tendency that makes sense for a nominal variable is the mode. The mean and median for nominal variables are not meaningful. Although you can get Stata or any other software program to produce a mean and a median for nominal variables, that doesn't mean they have any meaningful value.
- There are lots of nominal-type characteristics that are important predictors of the things that social scientists are interested in – but because we can't determine a 'meaningful mean' or median, we need to make a special adjustment so that we can use nominal variables in multivariate statistics.

See Box 3.2 if you've heard of dummy variables but aren't exactly sure what they are or how to interpret them.

Box 3.2: Dummy variables

Let us start with a typical dummy variable: sex. Sex is a nominal variable and a predictor of many dependent variables in which we are interested: pay, poverty, family structure, etc. But sex is nominal, which limits what we can do with it in terms of statistics. However, there are ways of including nominal variables in statistical analysis through the use of these dummy variables. If we take the example of sex, a transformation into a dummy variable would mean that we would pick one (category of) sex and code it 1 (e.g. female), leaving the other sex (in this case, male) to be coded 0. Why would we do this?

Let's look at it in a spreadsheet:

ID	Sex (1 = female)
1	1
2	1
3	0
4	0
5	0
6	1
7	1
8	0
9	1
10	1

In this example, ID just refers to the personal identifier of the respondent, and sex is the dummy variable, where 1 = female and 0 = male. When we transform our variable into a dummy variable like this, it becomes possible to calculate a mean that we can interpret. If we add up the values of the variable sex above and divide by the number of cases, we get:

$$(1 + 1 + 0 + 0 + 0 + 1 + 1 + 0 + 1 + 0)/10 = 0.6$$

Because we've transformed the variable into 1s and 0s, what this number represents now is the proportion of the sample that takes the value 1 on the dummy variable; that is, the proportion of the sample that is female. So typically, you would see a dummy variable such as this presented in a table of descriptive statistics like this:

Variable	Mean	Standard Dev.	Minimum	Maximum
Sex (1 = female)	0.6	–	0	1

Sometimes the note '(1 = female)' isn't presented and the authors just put 'Female' instead of 'Sex' as the variable name, assuming that readers will understand that it is dummy variable:

Variable	Mean	Standard Dev.	Minimum	Maximum
Female	0.6	–	0	1

So, both of these examples mean exactly the same thing: 60% of the sample is female. There is also the additional hint that the variable is a 'dummy' because the minimum is reported as 0 and the maximum is reported as 1. The standard deviation for dummy variables is not interpretable, although some authors occasionally put it in.

Often, dummy variables are created out of yes/no questionnaire items as well (which are also dichotomous). Suppose you saw something like this:

Variable	Mean	Standard Dev.	Minimum	Maximum
Capital punishment should be reinstated	0.15	–	0	1
Single parent	0.45	–	0	1

▶

▶ You could understand it to mean that 15% of the sample answered 'Yes' to a questionnaire item which asked if they think capital punishment should be reinstated. Similarly, 45% of this sample were single parents when the only possible categories in the variable were 1 = yes, 0 = no.

Nominal variables with more than two categories

Nominal variables often have more than two categories. Let us consider the example of a measure of where people live or their region of residence with a variable that has the following categories: 1= North, 2 = South, 3 = East, 4 = West. If you want to include region as an independent variable in your study you need to make some adjustments to it. You must make dummy variables for as many categories as there are in the original variable. In other words, we need to make four dummy variables to measure region in this example. So what we do is:

- make a variable *North* where 1 = North 0 = all other responses;
- make a variable *South* where 1 = South 0 = all other responses;
- make a variable *East* where 1 = East 0 = all other responses;
- make a variable *West* where 1 = West 0 = all other responses.

Let's look at our original variable in a spreadsheet:

ID	Region
1	3
2	2
3	4
4	1
5	1
6	1
7	2
8	3
9	2
10	2

So we have 3 cases in the North, 4 in the South, 2 in the East, and 1 in the West. When we convert region into dummy variables, the spreadsheet will look like this:

ID	Region	North	South	East	West
1	**3**	0	0	**1**	0
2	**2**	0	**1**	0	0
3	**4**	0	0	0	**1**
4	**1**	**1**	0	0	0
5	**1**	**1**	0	0	0
6	**1**	**1**	0	0	0
7	**2**	0	**1**	0	0
8	**3**	0	0	**1**	0
9	**2**	0	**1**	0	0
10	**2**	0	**1**	0	0

We have the original variable here and the four dummy variables. If we compute the mean of the dummy variables we will get:

North, $(0 + 0 + 0 + 1 + 1 + 1 + 0 + 0 + 0 + 0)/10 = 0.3$;
South, $(0 + 1 + 0 + 0 + 0 + 0 + 1 + 0 + 1 + 1)/10 = 0.4$;
East, $(1 + 0 + 0 + 0 + 0 + 0 + 0 + 1 + 0 + 0)/10 = 0.2$;
West, $(0 + 0 + 1 + 0 + 0 + 0 + 0 + 0 + 0 + 0 +)/10 = 0.1$.

These means represent the proportion of those who had the value 1 on each of the dummy variables. In a table, you would see this presented typically as:

Variable	Mean	Standard Dev	Minimum	Maximum
Region				
North	0.3	–	0	1
South	0.4	–	0	1
East	0.2	–	0	1
West	0.1	–	0	1

▶

▶ We have four dummy variables measuring region. Of our sample, 30% live in the North, 40% in the South, 20% in the East, and 10% in the West. Note that if you add up these percentages, you get 100%, and likewise if you add up the numbers in the 'mean' column, you will end up with 1.0.

You may wonder why the variable sex can be converted into just one dummy variable and region required four. The reason is that when we convert a dichotomous variable (which only has two categories in the original) we only need to present one variable for the category we choose to code as '1'. It is assumed that whatever the other category for the dichotomous variable was will be represented as the zero.

You will want to note that when you use dummy variables in a multivariate analysis, one group always is omitted as the 'reference category'. In the case of sex, male is omitted and the coefficients for 'female' would be compared to those for 'male'. In the example of region, one category would have to be omitted (e.g. North) and the other categories compared to the omitted category when interpreting the results. This will be discussed further when we are including dummy variables in multivariate estimations in Chapters 8 and 9.

As we've said before, and will say again, there is often more than one way to complete a task in Stata that gets you to the right answer. The creation of variables is a case in point. Let us show you some different ways of creating dummy variables.

Suppose we wanted to create a dummy variable for those who have a university degree called *degree* from the *educ* variable where there are 12 categories of qualifications, with 1 and 2 being degrees and the missing values recoded to a dot (.). We could do this in a number of more or less efficient ways.

(a)   Create a new variable and recode it:
```
generate degree1=educ
recode degree1 1/2=1 3/max=0
```

(b)   Recode *educ* and make the new variable at the same time:
```
recode educ (1/2=1) (3/max=0), ///
    gen (degree2)
```

(c) Use **generate** and **replace** commands:
```
gen degree3=1 if educ<=2
replace degree3=0 if educ>=3 & ///
    !missing(educ)
```

(d) Use the **generate** command in one line:
```
gen degree4=educ<=2 if !missing(educ)
```

It is very important in (c) and (d) to have the **!missing(educ)** element at the end – note that one is a **&** and the other is an **if**. If you make another variable (*degree5*) where you omit this part from (d), and then do a frequency distribution on both, you will see that they are different.

```
gen degree5=educ<=2
tab1 degree4 degree5
```

```
. tab1 degree4 degree5

-> tabulation of degree4

degree4 |     Freq.     Percent      Cum.
--------+-----------------------------------
      0 |     9,173       92.72      92.72
      1 |       720        7.28     100.00
--------+-----------------------------------
  Total |     9,893      100.00

-> tabulation of degree5

degree5 |     Freq.     Percent      Cum.
--------+-----------------------------------
      0 |     9,544       92.99      92.99
      1 |       720        7.01     100.00
--------+-----------------------------------
  Total |    10,264      100.00
```

Where have the missing values gone? Without the **!missing(educ)** element of the command, Stata has put all the missing values into the 0 category of the dummy variable *degree 5*. This is because Stata recognizes missing values (dot, .a, etc.) as a very high number and every time we use < or > we must ensure that we tell Stata not to include missing values!

You may wonder why, in (d), Stata knows to make a variable coded 1 and 0. Nowhere in the code are 0 and 1 explicitly stated, like in the other examples. This has to do with how Stata understands double and single equal signs. In (d), we are setting a condition and if it is met, Stata logically assigns 1 to the condition and 0 to the cases were the condition is not met. See Box 3.3 on double and single equal signs for more information on this topic.

Now we have created five variables measuring whether or not someone has a degree. We don't need all these. We can get rid of the redundant variables using the command **drop**.

```
drop degree1 degree2 degree3 degree5
```

Box 3.3: Single and double equals signs

New users to Stata often get confused as to when single (=) or double (==) equals signs should be used. A simple rule of thumb is that a single equals sign is used to assign the value at the right of it the value to the left. For example, in the command

```
generate x=educ
```

a new variable called *x* has been created which is the same as the variable *educ*. We have told Stata that *x* is going to be the same as *educ*.

A double equal sign, on the other hand, is used to check whether the value to the right is the same as the value to the left. It is used for comparison purposes, rather than 'assignment' (like the single equal sign). The command

```
summarize if sex==2
```

would return the summary statistics of all variables in the data set for females only.

So if you are going to set the values of a variable to something, use a single equals sign, and if you are testing for equality, use the double equals signs. As with anything else, the more you practice, the more it makes sense. Often, single and double equals signs are used within the same operation.

Often when we want to include nominal (categorical) variables in statistical estimations, it is necessary to create a series of dummy variables from the original variable. This is done easily by combining the **tab** and **gen** commands. For example, if we wanted to create a series of dummies for the job status variable:

```
tab jbstat, gen(jobstat)
```

If you look at the bottom of your variable list, you will see that a number of dummy variables have been created (*jobstat1*, *jobstat2*, *jobstat3*, etc.). You can do a frequency distribution of these variables like any other variable. You will see that they are all dichotomized into a 0/1 format.

LABELLING VARIABLES

From our previous example on page 50 we have a new marital status variable (*mastat2*). Having done the frequency distribution (**tab**) of the variable, we can see that there are no labels attached to the values of the variable. Now we want to label the variable and values so that we don't forget which each number stands for. Labeling in Stata is a bit different for those used to labeling variables in other statistical software packages. There are essentially three steps:

1. Create a label for the variable itself.
2. Define a label for values.
3. Attach that label to a specific variable.

We first label our variable:

```
label var mastat2 "simpler marital status"
```

Now our variable *mastat2* has a label 'simpler marital status'. If you **tab mastat2** you will see this new label and it will also be in your variable list.

Now we want to label the values of the categories of *mastat2*. To do this use the command **label define**. First, we have to define a name for our labels. We are calling these labels 'marital'.

```
lab def marital 1 "partnered" 2 "prev married" ///
    3 "single"
```

If you make an error when you are using this command and try to do it again, you will likely get a message that the labels have already been defined. Stata will not let you overwrite labels unless it is sure that you actually want to! You can assure Stata that you intend to overwrite labels by adding the option **modify**. Try:

lab def marital 1 "partnered" 2 "prev married" ///
**   3 "single", modify**

It is important to realize that at this point you have defined a label, but this label is not yet attached to any variable categories. The label exists separately from any variable. If you type **label list** you will see all the labels in your data set. The label for 'marital' will be there with all the category values defined as we have entered them above.

   Now we must attach these category labels to the variable using the procedure **label value**.

lab val mastat2 marital

This tells Stata to attach the values we assigned to the label 'marital' to the variable *mastat2*. Once value labels have been defined they can be applied to other variables. If we now tabulate the new marital status variable we get:

```
. ta mastat2

    simpler |
    marital |
     status |     Freq.    Percent       Cum.
------------+-----------------------------------
  partnered |     6,683      65.18      65.18
prev married |     1,489      14.52      79.70
     single |     2,081      20.30     100.00
------------+-----------------------------------
      Total |    10,253     100.00
```

This may seem like a nonsense way of doing labels, but it does have one really great benefit. If you have numerous variables with the same codes (e.g. 'yes' and 'no'), it is very easy to label them.

We have created some dummy variables earlier in the chapter: one for self-employed women and one for degrees. To label them all, we would just define a label:

```
lab def yesno 1 "yes" 0 "no"
```

and then attach these values to our dummy variables:

```
lab val fem1 yesno
lab val degree4 yesno
```
. . . etc

If you were using multiple dummy variables in your data set, you can easily see how quick it would be to label them all.

For ways of changing a number of variable names at once, see the commands in Box 3.4.

Box 3.4: Renaming variables

If a variable already has a name you might want to change it. It could be that the original one isn't as informative as it should be; some of the older data sets were very restricted in the number of characters they could use to name variables, so it's not uncommon to see variable names such as *sdt0068* for the number of children in the house which it would more convenient to change to *numchd*. For this example you would use:

```
rename sdt0068 numchd
```

The **rename** command is suitable when you only have a few variables to change as you can only change one variable per **rename** command. If you have more than half a dozen variables to change it is worth installing the **renvars** command. Type:

```
findit renvars
```

Then follow the instructions to install the command.   ▶

▶   There are a number of options with **renvars** but mostly it allows you to rename multiple variables in one command. Let's continue with our example above where a data set has variable names *std0068*, *std0069* and *std0070* and you want to change these to more meaningful names. Typing

```
renvars std0068 std0069 std0070 \ numchd ///
    chdage chdsex
```

would change the variable names listed to the left of the backslash (\) to the new variable names to the right of the backslash in the respective order. If the original variables are consecutive in the data set then you can just put the first and last separated by a dash (as with many other Stata commands), for example:

```
renvars std0068-std0070 \ numchd chdage chdsex
```

Another useful command to be aware of is **renpfix**. This command can either change variable name stubs, such as *sdt* in our example, or remove them completely. If you wanted to change *sdt* stub to *chd* for our three example variables, you would type

```
renpfix std chd
```

You would now have three variables: *chd0068*, *chd0069* and *chd0070*. If you typed

```
renpfix st
```

Stata would remove the *st* stub from all variables that start with that stub, in this case leaving three variables named *d0068*, *d0069* and *d0070*. All variables that start with the stub will be changed, so be careful with this command. Note that you cannot use variable names that start with a number.

A common use for **renpfix** is if you have panel data and each wave of data has variables that start with the same letter. In the British Household Panel Survey all the variables in the first wave start with *a*, second wave start with *b*, third wave start with *c*, and so on. When you put data sets together in a panel format the variables need to be named the same in each so **renpfix** can be used to remove the starting letter (stub) from all variable names.

MORE ON GENERATING NEW VARIABLES

Stata has a second, 'extended' generate command that allows you to create numerous types of variables from your existing data both for analysis and for data management. The command is **egen** and as you get more familiar with Stata then you will probably find yourself using this command more and more as it is very powerful. There are a considerable number of uses for **egen** so we cannot cover all of them here. Instead we use a few examples to illustrate its utility. Remember that you can type **help egen** to find out all of the ways to use the command.

The **group** function of **egen** creates a new variable by combining categories of two or more variables. Let's take a simple example of two variables both with only two categories. First we make a variable that indicates those who are married compared to all others:

```
recode mastat (1=1) (2/max=0), gen(married)
```

We have included the **(1=1)** for clarity but it is not strictly necessary for this recode. Now we want to create a new variable that has the following four categories: married men, married women, unmarried men, and unmarried women. If we crosstabulated the variables *married* and *sex* we would see that:

```
ta sex married
```

```
. ta sex married

         |  RECODE of mastat
         |  (marital status)
    sex  |         0          1 |     Total
---------+----------------------+----------
   male  |     1,886      2,947 |     4,833
 female  |     2,369      3,062 |     5,431
---------+----------------------+----------
  Total  |     4,255      6,009 |    10,264
```

From this table we can see the numbers in each of the four categories we are interested in, but we don't have them in a single variable. The long way to do this would be to use the **gen** and **replace** commands with **if** statements such as:

```
gen sexmar1=1 if sex==1&married==0
replace sexmar1=2 if sex==1&married==1
replace sexmar1=3 if sex==2&married==0
replace sexmar1=4 if sex==2&married==1
```

```
. gen sexmar1=1 if sex==1&married==0
(8378 missing values generated)

. replace sexmar1=2 if sex==1&married==1
(2947 real changes made)

. replace sexmar1=3 if sex==2&married==0
(2369 real changes made)

. replace sexmar1=4 if sex==2&married==1
(3062 real changes made)
```

Then if we label the categories and tabulate the new variable:

```
lab def sexmar 1 "unmarried men" ///
   2 "married men" 3 "unmarried women" ///
   4 "married women"
lab val sexmar1 sexmar
ta sexmar1
```

```
. lab def sexmar 1 "unmarried men" ///
   2 "married men" 3 "unmarried women" ///
   4 "married women"

. lab val sexmar1 sexmar

. ta sexmar1

        sexmar1 |     Freq.    Percent       Cum.
----------------+---------------------------------
  unmarried men |     1,886      18.37      18.37
    married men |     2,947      28.71      47.09
unmarried women |     2,369      23.08      70.17
  married women |     3,062      29.83     100.00
----------------+---------------------------------
          Total |    10,264     100.00
```

If you compare the categories of this new variable with the crosstabulation of *sex* and *married* above you can see the new categories represent each cell of the crosstabulation. However, using the **egen** command considerably shortens this process:

```
egen sexmar2=group(sex married)
ta sexmar2
```

```
. ta sexmar2
```

group(sex married)	Freq.	Percent	Cum.
1	1,886	18.37	18.37
2	2,947	28.71	47.09
3	2,369	23.08	70.17
4	3,062	29.83	100.00
Total	10,264	100.00	

We ordered our **replace** commands to re-create the process that the **egen group** command uses to make its categories so that you can easily compare the results. This is that the first category of the first variable in the list is taken first and then groups are made with that and the categories of the second variable. So, in the *sex* variable 1 = men and 2 = women, and in the *married* variable 0 = unmarried and 1 = married. Therefore the categories of the new variable are 1 = men unmarried, 2 = men married, 3 = women unmarried, 4 = women married. So we can use the label 'sexmar' with this variable as well:

```
lab val sexmar2 sexmar
ta sexmar2
```

```
. ta sexmar2
```

group(sex married)	Freq.	Percent	Cum.
unmarried men	1,886	18.37	18.37
married men	2,947	28.71	47.09
unmarried women	2,369	23.08	70.17
married women	3,062	29.83	100.00
Total	10,264	100.00	

Obviously, this gets more complicated if the variables have more than two categories and if you use more than two variables. It's important to understand how Stata orders categories of variables in a list; not only for this command but for many others as well such as the **by** and **bysort** commands that we cover in Chapter 4.

The second function of **egen** we cover here is **rownonmiss**. This function tells Stata to look across a number of variables and, for each case (row), create a new variable that shows how many non-missing values there are. Non-missing means any value which has not being designated as missing (. or .a, .b, etc.). Remember that you need to have coded the values to missing prior to using this command. In this example, we take three General Health Questionnaire (GHQ) items, *ghqa*, *ghqb* and *ghqd*, to show how this command works by creating a new variable called *obs*. Then to show the frequencies of the new variable we need to tabulate it:

```
egen obs=rownonmiss(ghqa ghqb ghqd)
ta obs
```

```
. egen obs=rownonmiss(ghqa ghqb ghqd)

. ta obs
```

obs	Freq.	Percent	Cum.
0	530	5.16	5.16
1	1	0.01	5.17
2	14	0.14	5.31
3	9,719	94.69	100.00
Total	10,264	100.00	

This table shows us that 9719 people answered all three questions, 14 answered two (note that this doesn't show you which two), 1 answered only one question, and 530 did not answer any of the three questions. Another way of looking at this is that those given a zero on the variable *obs* are missing on all three questions. To show this, we tabulate the three variables for those who have a zero:

```
tab1 ghqa ghqb ghqd if obs==0
```

```
. tab1 ghqa ghqb ghqd if obs==0

-> tabulation of ghqa if obs==0
no observations
```

```
-> tabulation of ghqb if obs==0
no observations

-> tabulation of ghqd if obs==0
no observations
```

This confirms that those 530 cases have not answered any of the three questions.

The values of *obs* can be used in a number of ways when creating and manipulating variables, especially when creating scales (see below) and deciding how many questions need to be answered to be included. It may also be used to select cases for analysis or to manage data sets when some cases are kept or dropped.

We carry on using the three GHQ items to demonstrate another function of **egen**. This function, **rowmean**, creates a new variable with a value of the mean of the variables specified. The default method for this function creates a mean for any cases that have at least one non-missing value. So, a mean might be created for someone who has only answered one of the questions. You need to decide if that is something you wish to do. So, we will use the *obs* variable created by the **rownonmiss** function to refine the variable creation. We start with the default method:

egen mean1=rowmean(ghqa ghqb ghqd)

```
. egen mean1=rowmean(ghqa ghqb ghqd)
(530 missing values generated)
```

Stata tells us that the new variable, *mean1*, has been created with 530 missing values. Refer back to the table of *obs* and see that 530 cases were missing on all three questions and these are the ones that are missing on this new variable. While you are looking at the table of *obs*, you can see that one person answered only one of the three questions. If we wanted to exclude that person from having a mean then we can use the values of *obs* to condition the **rowmean** function by restricting it to only those who answered two or three questions:

egen mean2=rowmean(ghqa ghqb ghqd) if obs>1

```
. egen mean2=rowmean(ghqa ghqb ghqd)if obs>1
(531 missing values generated)
```

The output shows 531 missing values in the new variable, *mean2*, which reflects the inclusion of the person who only answered one question. To follow this example through to its logical conclusion we now use the **rowmean** function and the values of the *obs* variable to calculate a mean for only those who answered all three questions:

egen mean3=rowmean(ghqa ghqb ghqd) if obs==3

```
. egen mean3=rowmean(ghqa ghqb ghqd) if obs==3
(545 missing values generated)
```

Now for the new variable, *mean3*, there are 545 missing values, 14 more than in *mean2*, which shows that the 14 people who only answered two questions are now given missing values. We now show the descriptives of all three newly created mean value variables:

su mean*

```
. su mean*

Variable |     Obs        Mean   Std. Dev.   Min   Max
---------+-------------------------------------------------
   mean1 |    9734    1.976645    .4311008     1     4
   mean2 |    9733    1.976643    .4311229     1     4
   mean3 |    9719    1.976198    .4302754     1     4
```

This output shows the different number of non-missing observations in each of the mean score variables. The relatively small number of cases that did not answer all three questions means that their exclusion has very little effect on the mean scores for the sample. However, there are other reasons why you may want to exclude these cases or you may be happy to include them.

CREATING A SCALE

It is often useful to create a scale out of a number of variables in a data set to measure a more general concept. You may, for example, have 10 different variables that measure depression, but find that they can be grouped together to form a single overall measure of depression. There are, mathematically, many ways to create a scale, but one common way is to simply add up the variables to create a summed scale.

We have a number of GHQ (Goldberg and Williams 1988) measures in our sample data set. If we add these up and create a summed measure, we would do it like this:

```
gen ghq= ghqa+ ghqb+ ghqc+ ghqd+ ghqe+ ///
    ghqf+ ghqg+ ghqh+ ghqi+ ghqj+ ghqk+ ghql
```

This command might look a little cumbersome, so let's use the **egen** command to do the same thing:

```
egen obs2=rownonmiss(ghqa-ghql)
egen ghq2=rowtotal(ghqa-ghql) if obs==12
```

Compare the two:

```
su ghq ghq2
```

```
. su ghq ghq2

Variable |    Obs        Mean   Std. Dev.   Min    Max
---------+---------------------------------------------
    ghq |   9613    22.77125    4.914182     12     48
   ghq2 |   9613    22.77125    4.914182     12     48
```

Be careful how you use the **rowtotal** function in **egen** as it does different things with missing values in some circumstances between version 9 and 10, so it would be best to check using **help egen**. In this example it's not a problem as we are using the *obs2* variable to determine which cases to add across the variables.

The variables used to make up this scale all have values from 1 to 4 with high values that are associated with an undesirable characteristic, such as being depressed, being under strain, or having lessened ability to face problems. So the resulting scale has a minimum of 12 and a maximum of 48. You should note that individuals who are missing on even one of the composite items are given a 'missing' value in the overall scale because of the condition **obs2==12**.

The GHQ is a well-established scale and we can be fairly confident of its reliability and validity. But what if we are working with data that are less familiar?

It is very important that you are familiar with the variables in your proposed scale and that they are all in the 'same direction'.

The difference between Stata and other statistical software programs is that if you were making a satisfaction scale in SPSS, for example, it would be important that all the variables used to create this scale all have the same 'direction' of measurement. If some are coded in the opposite order (to measure dissatisfaction, for example), you would have to recode these items so that all the measures were in the same direction (i.e. measuring the extent of satisfaction). Stata, however, has the ability to examine variables and 'reverse score' items that it thinks are reverse coded using the command **alpha**. The default setting in Stata is to empirically determine the relationship and reverse the scorings for any that enter (i.e. are correlated with other items) negatively. We will return to this topic shortly.

But how do you know if it is a good scale? There are several ways of assessing the reliability of a scale. One of the most common is the Cronbach's alpha, which is what the scaling command **alpha** is based upon. For all proposed scale items, **alpha** computes the inter-item correlations (or covariances) for all pairs of variables in the variable list. The command will also return a Cronbach's alpha statistic for the new scale. Cronbach's alpha statistic ranges from 0 to 1, with values closer to one indicating a 'better', more internally consistent scale. It should be noted, however, that scales comprised of a high number of variables will have higher alpha values than scales with the same inter-item correlations but with fewer variables. So the number of items in a scale must be kept in mind when assessing alpha value. However, in general, a value of about 0.70 or higher is generally considered acceptable for a scale.

Let's try a different set of variables – those that assess opinions on women and their role in the home and workplace. To find out how good our measure is, we can ask Stata to report a reliability coefficient for us:

```
alpha opfama opfamb opfamc opfamd opfame ///
    opfamf opfamg opfamh opfami
```

or

```
alpha opfama-opfami
```

Note that if you use the latter of these two **alpha** commands, the variables must be in this order in your variable list.

```
. alpha opfama-opfami

Test scale = mean(unstandardized items)
Reversed items: opfamc opfamd opfame opfamh
opfami

Average interitem covariance:      .204454
Number of items in the scale:            9
Scale reliability coefficient:      0.6958
```

We are given an alpha of 0.6958, which is a little on the low side for a nine-item scale. We can also see that Stata has listed a number of reversed items. This means that Stata has decided that these five items are 'negatively' scored compared to the other items in the scale, and as such, has 'reverse coded' them to fit in with the theme of the scale.

Let's examine the items as they were asked to the survey respondents.

opfama: A pre-school child is likely to suffer if his or her mother works.

opfamb: All in all, family life suffers when the woman has a full-time job.

opfamc: A woman and her family would all be happier if she goes out to work.

opfamd: Both the husband and wife should both contribute to the household income.

opfame: Having a full-time job is the best way for a woman to be an independent person.

opfamf: A husband's job is to earn money; a wife's job is to look after the home and family.

opfamg: Children need a father to be as closely involved in their upbringing as the mother.

opfamh: Employers should make special arrangements to help mothers combine jobs and childcare.

opfami: A single parent can bring up children as well as a couple.

The response categories for all items were: (1) strongly agree, (2) agree, (3) neither agree nor disagree, (4) disagree and (5) strongly disagree.

As the items are, if a person strongly agreed that pre-school children suffered if a mother worked (*opfama*), he or she would get a score of 1. However, such a person would be unlikely to strongly agree with the statement that a woman and her family would be happier if she worked (*opfamc*). In this case, the respondent might strongly disagree with such a statement, giving a score of 5. However, both these opinions reflect a tendency to be 'conservative' in opinions about gender roles in a family. Stata has picked up that people who answered in certain ways on items like *opfama* and *opfamb* (where high scores reflect more 'liberal' opinions about gender roles) were likely to have 'reversed' scores on items *opfamc, opfamd, opfame, opfamh*, and *opfami* (where high scores reflect a more 'conservative' orientation). As the items that were 'reverse scored' were more conservative, this means that higher scores on our new scale are associated with more liberal opinions.

But does Stata always get it right? It is the case that the five items highlighted by Stata as being reverse coded are 'opposite' in direction to *opfama, opfamb*, and *opfamf*. But you could argue that agreeing with *opfamg* may also indicate more liberal views. Stata, however, hasn't picked this up.

The problem isn't something with Stata. The algorithm with which Stata works to decide which items should be reverse coded relies on the item's correlations with the other scale items. If it is negatively correlated, it becomes reverse coded.

Let's create a correlation matrix of these items:

```
. corr opfam*
(obs=9510)

        |  opfama  opfamb  opfamc  opfamd  opfame  opfamf  opfamg opfamh opfami
--------+-----------------------------------------------------------------------------
opfama  |  1.0000
opfamb  |  0.6465  1.0000
opfamc  | -0.2798 -0.3550  1.0000
opfamd  | -0.1230 -0.1620  0.3192  1.0000
opfame  | -0.1059 -0.1797  0.3327  0.3610  1.0000
opfamf  |  0.4375  0.5438 -0.2455 -0.1043 -0.0756  1.0000
opfamg  |  0.1456  0.1215 -0.0225  0.0883  0.0496  0.0959  1.0000
opfamh  | -0.1892 -0.1825  0.1746  0.1729  0.1606 -0.2193  0.1356 1.0000
opfami  | -0.2871 -0.2698  0.1406  0.1312  0.0860 -0.1895 -0.1476 0.2153 1.0000
```

You can see from this matrix that the reverse coded items (*opfamc, opfamd, opfame, opfamh, opfami*) are negatively correlated with *opfama, opfamb* and *opfamf* (and positively with the other 'reverse coded' items). On the other hand, *opfamg* does not follow this general pattern, which is why it wasn't reverse coded by Stata.

There are a couple possible reasons for this. The most likely is that it is not a good item for your scale – that it somehow does not 'fit' as well as the other items. You can check this by using the option **item**:

alpha opfama-opfami,item

```
. alpha opfama-opfami,item

Test scale = mean(unstandardized items)
```

Item	Obs	Sign	item-test correlation	item-rest correlation	average inter-item covariance	alpha
opfama	9628	+	0.6949	0.5465	.172436	0.6301
opfamb	9662	+	0.7466	0.6127	.1618418	0.6131
opfamc	9640	-	0.5667	0.4340	.2053443	0.6604
opfamd	9646	-	0.4510	0.2786	.2201311	0.6863
opfame	9648	-	0.4481	0.2639	.2198141	0.6896
opfamf	9652	+	0.6375	0.4588	.1808333	0.6498
opfamg	9657	+	0.2283	0.0726	.2533817	0.7152
opfamh	9645	-	0.4424	0.2746	.2222064	0.6866
opfami	9648	-	0.5297	0.3319	.2040992	0.6788
Test scale					.204454	0.6958

Of particular interest is the last column labelled 'alpha'. It would be better labelled as 'alpha if item removed', because that is what it is telling us. If we look down to *opfamg*, we can see that the alpha of the scale would improve to 0.7152 if we took this item out. Alpha can only tell us this information for items one at a time – it won't tell us the effect on alpha of removing two or three items at once.

So it seems that *opfamg* isn't such a great measure for our proposed scale. And if we look at it, we can see that the item is somewhat different from the other items because it is asking about general child upbringing, rather than issues pertaining specifically to employment.

It should be stressed that you should always check the items in your scale and make sure that they make theoretical sense. The mathematical techniques involved in scale construction do not do this for you!

So what happens if we take out *opfamg*?

```
. alpha opfama opfamb opfamc opfamd opfame opfamf opfamh ///
    opfami,item

Test scale = mean(unstandardized items)
```

Item	Obs	Sign	item-test correlation	item-rest correlation	average inter-item covariance	alpha
opfama	9628	+	0.6880	0.5338	.2231625	0.6574
opfamb	9662	+	0.7448	0.6076	.2081992	0.6384
opfamc	9640	−	0.5771	0.4419	.2618421	0.6824
opfamd	9646	−	0.4773	0.3036	.2777641	0.7062
opfame	9648	−	0.4684	0.2815	.2786443	0.7112
opfamf	9652	+	0.6393	0.4534	.2327838	0.6764
opfamh	9645	−	0.4754	0.3076	.2790421	0.7050
opfami	9648	−	0.5191	0.3129	.2656042	0.7083
Test scale					.2533817	0.7152

We can see that the alpha has improved and that no further removal of individual items will increase our alpha.

As we haven't created the scale variable yet, we could ask Stata to create it for us after it computed the reliability using the **gen** option.

```
alpha opfama opfamb opfamc opfamd opfame ///
    opfamf opfamh opfami, gen(famscale1)
```

The **gen** option tells Stata to create a new variable (we have named it *famscale1*). Unless we tell Stata otherwise, it will go ahead and reverse code items. If you are ever in a position where you don't want Stata to do this, typing the option **asis** will tell Stata not to reverse code any items. You can also use the option **std** to get Stata to create the new variable in standardized form (a mean of 0 and a standard deviation of 1).

It is very important to note how Stata handles missing data in the **alpha** command. In other commands that we have talked about so far in this book, cases are deleted from the analysis if they are missing on at least one of the variables under consideration. So when we **tab sex age**, if a case is missing on the age variable, it will not be included in the tabulation. It is deleted 'casewise'. Similarly, we could create the scale just by simply adding up all the variables using the **gen** command (after reverse coding manually). Now, the cases where there was missing data on one or more of the scale items would not be included. The default in the **gen** option, however, is to create a score for every observation where there is a response to at least one scale item. In other words, a scale value could be created for someone who answered only one of the eight *opfam* variables. The score is calculated by dividing the summative score over the total number of items available for the specific case.

If you find this objectionable (we do!), you may want to employ the option **casewise** so that cases with any missing values on the scale items are deleted. Let's see how this changes our results.

```
alpha opfama opfamb opfamc opfamd opfame ///
    opfamf opfamh opfami,gen(famscale2) casewise
```

```
. alpha opfama opfamb opfamc opfamd opfame ///
    opfamf opfamh opfami,gen(famscale2) casewise

Test scale = mean(unstandardized items)
Reversed items: opfamc opfamd opfame opfamh
    opfami

Average interitem covariance:      .2540916
Number of items in the scale:             8
Scale reliability coefficient:       0.7166
```

The results suggest a slightly better alpha. But we also know that cases are only included if respondents answered all the items in our scale.

If you don't want to be so stringent, you can set an alternative minimum number of items that must be non-missing in order for the scale to be constructed. Let's say we decided that a person must have answered at least five of the eight items in order to be included in the scale, we would use the option **min**.

```
alpha opfama opfamb opfamc opfamd opfame ///
    opfamf opfamh opfami, gen(famscale3) min(5)
```

When we create a scale, we are just really adding up items and, as such, we would rightly expect that if we are adding up 8 items, all of which have values of 1 to 5, our scale will have a minimum of 8 and a maximum of 40. People who score 8 would be very conservative, while those around the 40 mark would be rather liberal.

```
recode opfamc opfamd opfame opfamh opfami ///
    (1=5) (2=4) (3=3) (4=2) (5=1)
```

```
gen famscale4= opfama+ opfamb+ opfamc+ ///
    opfamd+ opfame+ opfamf+ opfamh+ opfami
```

However, if we **summarize** our new variables (*famscale1*, *famscale2* and *famscale3*) and compare them with *famscale4* created by manually reverse coding and using **gen** to add the items (note the use of the wildcard * that saves typing all the variables). We get:

```
. su famscale*

    Variable |      Obs        Mean   Std. Dev.      Min    Max
-------------+-------------------------------------------------
   famscale1 |     9718   -.5544141    .6009038       -4      2
   famscale2 |     9515   -.5526143    .5954785    -2.75   1.25
   famscale3 |     9657   -.5529802    .5968845    -2.75      2
   famscale4 |     9515    25.57909    4.763828        8     40
```

What is happening?

In order to understand these values, you need to understand how Stata constructs the scale with the **alpha** command. When an item is 'reverse scored' it isn't recoded so that 1 becomes 5, 2 becomes 4, etc. What happens is that a negative sign is placed in front of all the original values so that the original values are changed to:

Variable	Direction	New values
opfama	+	1 2 3 4 5
opfamb	+	1 2 3 4 5
opfamc	–	–5 –4 –3 –2 –1
opfamd	–	–5 –4 –3 –2 –1
opfame	–	–5 –4 –3 –2 –1
opfamf	+	1 2 3 4 5
opfamh	–	–5 –4 –3 –2 –1
opfami	–	–5 –4 –3 –2 –1

This logic produces an overall total, for those who answered all eight items, with a minimum of −22 and a maximum of 10. If we divide these scores by 8 (the total number of items), we get −2.75 and 1.25 which match the minimum and maximum values in the data shown for *famscale2* which used the **casewise** option so that only cases with data on all eight items were included.

The theoretical minimum and maximum values for *famscale1*, created using the default settings for the **gen** option, are −5 and 5 as it is possible for respondents to answer just one item and be included in the scale. You can see from the Obs column that there are about 200 more cases in the *famscale1* variable than in the *famscale2* variable.

Determining the theoretical minimum and maximum values of the scale is a little more complex for *famscale3*, which used the option **min(5)** to tell Stata to use only cases that have answers to five or more items. If we take the five lowest possible scores which are the five reverse coded items then we get −25/5 = −5 as a minimum. The five highest possible scores are the three unaltered items and two reverse coded items: 5+5+5−1−1 so 13/5 = 2.6 is the maximum. You can see that the actual minimum and maximum values in the data fall short of these extremes.

However, if we correlate all four scales we see that they are mathematically equivalent for the cases that were included on each pair of scales. The decision rests with you, as the analyst, as to how many answers you need for someone to obtain an overall scale score.

```
. pwcorr famscale*,obs

           |  famsca~1   famsca~2   famsca~3   famsca~4
-----------+--------------------------------------------
 famscale1 |    1.0000
           |      9718
 famscale2 |    1.0000     1.0000
           |      9515       9515
 famscale3 |    1.0000     1.0000     1.0000
           |      9657       9515       9657
 famscale4 |    1.0000     1.0000     1.0000     1.0000
           |      9515       9515       9515       9515
```

For an account of using a scale in an applied research project, see Box 3.5.

Box 3.5: An example of using a scale in a project

In a project funded by the Department of Health we conducted a series of analyses investigating the consequences of early child-bearing on outcomes later in life. These were later published as papers examining housing,[1] partners and partnerships,[2] and gender differences in outcomes.[3] The data we used were from the British Cohort Study of 1970 which has followed approximately 15,000 children from birth in 1970 until the present day. Part of the analysis was to construct a measure of childhood behaviour prior to any childbearing. The cohort was interviewed at age 10 in 1980. At this time their teachers were also asked about their behaviour in school. We decided to use teacher reported behaviour as well as parent reported behaviour. We took all the answers from the teachers and examined the correlations between the variables and, after some thought and analysis, settled on a scale of five items that measured the child's concentration on educational tasks, their popularity with peers, the number of friends, their level of co-operation with peers, and the extent that the teachers were able to negotiate with the child. All items were measured using a 'thermometer' type response ranging from 1 to 47.

These five items had correlations between 0.33 and 0.84, which suggested that they might make a reasonable scale without all measuring the same thing. We standardized all five items to a mean of 0 and a standard deviation of 1 using the **egen** command to make five new variables: *zone, ztwo, zthree, zfour, zfive*. Then we used the **alpha** command to determine that the resulting scale had a Cronbach's alpha of 0.82, which was very satisfactory for a five-item scale. We used the **item** option on the **alpha** command to see if omitting items would improve the alpha value, and the results indicated that no significant improvement could be gained. To create the final score for each child we used the **egen**

---

[1] Ermisch, J.F. and Pevalin, D.J. (2004) Early childbearing and housing choices. *Journal of Housing Economics*, 13: 170–194.
[2] Ermisch, J.F. and Pevalin, D.J. (2005) Early motherhood and later partnerships. *Journal of Population Economics*, 18: 469–489.
[3] Robson, K. and Pevalin, D.J. (2007) Gender differences in the predictors and outcomes of young parenthood. *Research in Social Stratification and Mobility*, 25: 205–218.

command again to take a mean of the five items where a low score indicated poor behaviour.

```
. alpha zone- zfive,item

Test scale = mean(unstandardized items)

                                              average
                           item-test    item-rest inter-item
Item        |  Obs Sign correlation correlation covariance  alpha
------------+----------------------------------------------------
zone        | 12550   +      0.6689       0.4770  .5438279 0.8266
ztwo        | 12606   +      0.8546       0.7514  .4237435 0.7463
zthree      | 12575   +      0.8186       0.6949  .4474017 0.7641
zfour       | 12565   +      0.8164       0.6919  .4489863 0.7652
zfive       | 12506   +      0.6714       0.4816  .5412759 0.8252
------------+----------------------------------------------------
Test scale  |                                     .481128 0.8226
----------------------------------------------------------------
```

The final measure of childhood behaviour was a significant predictor of early parenthood, but the regression models indicated an interaction effect with gender (see Chapters 8 and 9 for regression and interaction effects) where this behaviour predicted early motherhood but not early fatherhood. Then we looked at when the cohort was 30 years old and we found that this behaviour measure was significantly associated with a range of outcomes including their educational attainment, labour force participation, pay, social class, house ownership, and receipt of benefits.

DEMONSTRATION EXERCISE

In this demonstration exercise we use some of the techniques covered in this and each of the subsequent chapters to conduct a series of data analyses exploring the question of social variations in mental health among working age adults. Our measure of mental health is the 12-item General Health Questionnaire, which is a scale that can be constructed in a number of ways. In this demonstration we start by using the GHQ in the form of a scale that ranges from 0 to 36, with higher scores indicating poorer mental health. The factors we are interested in using are sex, age, marital status, employment status, number of own children in the household and region of the country.

We start by opening the example data file (exampledata.dta) from our default directory. Before opening the data file we increase the memory available to Stata to 50 Mb using the **set mem** command:

```
version 10
set mem 50m
cd "C:\project folder"
use exampledata.dta
```

Next we use the **keep** command to retain only the individual level variables we need for this analysis and then recode all the negative values to missing. We keep the individual identifier (*pid*) and the household identifier (*hid*) so that we can match on household level information in the next chapter.

```
keep pid hid ghq* sex age mastat jbstat nchild
mvdecode _all,mv(-9/-1)
```

Stata returns the output below. You can see that after the **mvdecode** command, Stata tells you how many missing values were assigned for each variable. For example, the variable *jbstat* had 352 missing values while the variable *ghql* had 580 missing values. From this you can deduce that the variables *pid*, *hid*, *sex*, *age*, *mastat* and *nchild* do not have any missing values.

```
. mvdecode _all,mv(-9/-1)
       jbstat: 352 missing values generated
         ghqa: 536 missing values generated
         ghqb: 536 missing values generated
         ghqc: 545 missing values generated
         ghqd: 534 missing values generated
         ghqe: 535 missing values generated
         ghqf: 546 missing values generated
         ghqg: 534 missing values generated
         ghqh: 532 missing values generated
         ghqi: 534 missing values generated
         ghqj: 577 missing values generated
         ghqk: 587 missing values generated
         ghql: 580 missing values generated
```

We now create the GHQ scale from the 12 items in the data set. The items are coded from 1 to 4 but we want to make a scale that goes from 0 to 36, so we need to recode all the 12 GHQ items to go from 0 to 3. Note the use of the wildcard (*) to save listing every item. Another way to do this would be to use the dash as the items are in order in the data set (i.e. **recode ghqa-ghql**). We then check the internal consistency of the scale using the **alpha** command. In this example we use the **item** option to give us some more information.

```
recode ghq* (4=3) (3=2) (2=1) (1=0)
alpha ghq*,item
```

The output shows the changes made to each of the GHQ items then the details of the scale internal reliability check. The overall alpha value (0.8631) is reported at the bottom right of the table; all the signs are positive and all items have similar item–rest correlations. The right-hand column shows that the overall alpha value would not be increased by dropping any item. We should be reasonably happy with the internal reliability of this scale.

```
. recode ghq* (4=3) (3=2) (2=1) (1=0)
(ghqa: 9728 changes made)
(ghqb: 9728 changes made)
(ghqc: 9719 changes made)
(ghqd: 9730 changes made)
(ghqe: 9729 changes made)
(ghqf: 9718 changes made)
(ghqg: 9730 changes made)
(ghqh: 9732 changes made)
(ghqi: 9730 changes made)
(ghqj: 9687 changes made)
(ghqk: 9677 changes made)
(ghql: 9684 changes made)

. alpha ghq*,item
Test scale = mean(unstandardized items)
```

					average	
Item	Obs	Sign	item-test correlation	item-rest correlation	inter-item covariance	alpha
ghqa	9728	+	0.5891	0.5119	.1517366	0.8548
ghqb	9728	+	0.6413	0.5325	.1408634	0.8541
ghqc	9719	+	0.5092	0.4116	.1539663	0.8603
ghqd	9730	+	0.4798	0.3983	.1580361	0.8607
ghqe	9729	+	0.6981	0.5990	.1361276	0.8489
ghqf	9718	+	0.6835	0.5943	.1403709	0.8489
ghqg	9730	+	0.6220	0.5429	.1487009	0.8527
ghqh	9732	+	0.5680	0.4970	.154532	0.8561
ghqi	9730	+	0.7721	0.6895	.1299578	0.8415
ghqj	9687	+	0.7324	0.6497	.135947	0.8447
ghqk	9677	+	0.6483	0.5638	.1450927	0.8511
ghql	9684	+	0.6220	0.5479	.1499576	0.8528
Test scale					.1454405	0.8631

The command creates the scale using the **gen** command. As we have shown in this chapter, you could use the **alpha** command with a **gen** option but we prefer to construct the scale manually in this example.

```
gen ghqscale=ghqa+ghqb+ghqc+ghqd+ghqe+ghqf ///
   +ghqg+ghqh+ghqi+ghqj+ghqk+ghql
lab var ghqscale "ghq 0-36"
su ghqscale
```

In this part of the output, Stata lets us know that in creating the scale 651 missing values have been generated in the new variable (*ghqscale*). This is because the **gen** command only creates a new variable for those cases that have non-missing values on all 12 items. The next line labels the new variable and then we use the **su** command to display the descriptive statistics of the new variable, which shows that we have 9613 cases with a new scale score. There is further discussion of descriptive statistics commands in Chapter 5.

```
. gen ghqscale = ghqa+ghqb+ghqc+ghqd+ghqe ///
>     +ghqf+ghqg+ghqh+ghqi+ghqj+ghqk+ghql
(651 missing values generated)

. lab var ghqscale "ghq 0-36"

. su ghqscale
```

Variable	Obs	Mean	Std. Dev.	Min	Max
ghqscale	9613	10.77125	4.914182	0	36

We now construct another variable based on the GHQ items. This one uses a coding of 0–0–1–1 for each of the items and then adds up the items to a maximum of 12. Then a threshold of 4 or more is used to make a dichotomous indicator. First we recode all the 12 GHQ items and then sum them to create a new variable called *d_ghq*.

```
recode ghq* (0/1=0) (2/3=1)
gen d_ghq=ghqa+ghqb+ghqc+ghqd+ghqe+ghqf ///
   +ghqg+ghqh+ghqi+ghqj+ghqk+ghql
ta d_ghq
```

```
. ta d_ghq

  d_ghq |      Freq.     Percent        Cum.
--------+---------------------------------
      0 |     4,933       51.32       51.32
      1 |     1,423       14.80       66.12
      2 |       873        9.08       75.20
      3 |       600        6.24       81.44
      4 |       447        4.65       86.09
      5 |       341        3.55       89.64
      6 |       260        2.70       92.34
      7 |       210        2.18       94.53
      8 |       162        1.69       96.21
      9 |       103        1.07       97.28
     10 |       112        1.17       98.45
     11 |        94        0.98       99.43
     12 |        55        0.57      100.00
--------+---------------------------------
  Total |     9,613      100.00
```

The tabulation shows us that the recode and summing have been done correctly. Now we recode the *d_ghq* variable into a dichotomous indicator where 1 equals those with a GHQ score of 4 or more:

recode d_ghq 0/3=0 4/12=1
ta d_ghq

```
. ta d_ghq

   d_ghq |      Freq.     Percent        Cum.
---------+---------------------------------
       0 |     7,829       81.44       81.44
       1 |     1,784       18.56      100.00
---------+---------------------------------
   Total |     9,613      100.00
```

The tabulation of the dichotomous GHQ indicator shows that 18.56% of the current cases in the data set are over the threshold.

As we are interested in variations of mental health for those aged 18 to 65, we use the **keep** command to retain only those cases within that age range. Compare this use of the **keep** command – keeping cases – with the other use earlier in this example when it was used to keep variables. Similarly, the **drop** command can be used to drop variables or cases depending on how the command is formatted. We then produce descriptive statistics of the *age* variable to see how many cases we have left in our data.

```
keep if age>=18 & age<=65
su age
```

The output shows how many cases (observations) are deleted from the data set after implementing the **keep** command. From the descriptive statistics for the variable *age*, we see that now we only have 8163 cases in our data. Remember that there are no missing cases in the *age* variable.

```
. keep if age>=18 & age<=65
(2101 observations deleted)

. su age

Variable |    Obs      Mean   Std. Dev.   Min   Max
---------+----------------------------------------
     age |   8163   39.32733   13.08993    18    65
```

Next we recode the *age* variable into three categories and use the **gen** option in the **recode** command to create a new variable called *agecat*. We then label the new variable and its categories. We then use the **tab** command to produce a frequency table of the new variable to check if our recode and labelling have come out correctly.

```
recode age (18/32=1) (33/50=2) ///
   (51/65=3),gen(agecat)
lab var agecat "age categories"
lab def agelab 1 "18-32 years" ///
   2 "33-50 years" 3 "51-65 years"
lab val agecat agelab
tab agecat
```

After the **recode** command, Stata tells us that there are 8163 (all cases) differences between the original variable *age* and the newly created variable *agecat*. As we numbered the categories of *agecat* 1, 2, and 3 and there is no one in the data under 18 years of age, it is not surprising that for all cases the values of *age* and *agecat* are different. The frequency table produced from the **tab** command shows the number and percentage of the cases in each of the three age categories.

```
. recode age (18/32=1) (33/50=2) ///
    (51/65=3),gen(agecat)
(8163 differences between age and agecat)

. lab var agecat "age categories"

. lab def agelab 1 "18-32 years" ///
    2 "33-50 years" 3 "51-65 years"

. lab val agecat agelab

. tab agecat

        age |
  categories |   Freq.    Percent      Cum.
-------------+---------------------------------
18-32 years |   2,956      36.21      36.21
33-50 years |   3,336      40.87      77.08
51-65 years |   1,871      22.92     100.00
-------------+---------------------------------
      Total |   8,163     100.00
```

Our next step is to recode the *sex* variable into a dummy variable that indicates female cases. We use the **recode** command with the **gen** option again. We label the new variable and its categories, then produce a frequency table to check our recode.

```
tab sex
tab sex,nol
recode sex (1=0) (2=1),gen(female)
lab var female "female indicator"
lab def sexlab 0 "male" 1 "female"
lab val female sexlab
tab female
```

We see the frequency table of the *sex* variable but we need to see what numbers lie underneath the category labels of male and female. We use the **tab** command with the **nol** option.

```
. ta sex

      sex |     Freq.     Percent        Cum.
----------+-----------------------------------
     male |     3,914       47.95       47.95
   female |     4,249       52.05      100.00
----------+-----------------------------------
    Total |     8,163      100.00

. ta sex,nol

      sex |     Freq.     Percent        Cum.
----------+-----------------------------------
        1 |     3,914       47.95       47.95
        2 |     4,249       52.05      100.00
----------+-----------------------------------
    Total |     8,163      100.00

. recode sex (1=0) (2=1),gen(female)
(8163 differences between sex and female)

. lab var female "female indicator"

. lab def sexlab 0 "male" 1 "female"

. lab val female sexlab

. ta female

   female |
indicator |     Freq.     Percent        Cum.
----------+-----------------------------------
     male |     3,914       47.95       47.95
   female |     4,249       52.05      100.00
----------+-----------------------------------
    Total |     8,163      100.00
```

To reduce the number of marital status categories, we recode the marital status variable (*mastat*) into a new variable called *marst2* and have four categories, where 1 = single, 2 = married/cohabiting, 3 = separated/divorced and 4 = widowed. We need to see what the categories and the numbering are in the original marital status variable (*mastat*). We do this by using the **tab** command with the **nol** option. We then recode, create the new variable and label the new variable and its categories.

```
tab mastat
tab mastat,nol
recode mastat (6=1) (1/2=2) (4/5=3) ///
   (3=4),gen(marst2)
lab var marst2 "marital status 4 categories"
lab def marlab 1 "single" 2 "married" ///
   3 "sep/div" 4 "widowed"
lab val marst2 marlab
tab marst2
```

The output for these commands is similar to that above. The exact process and commands you use to recode variables may vary from this, but we strongly advise you to have a system that allows you to check your recoding as you go along.

```
. tab mastat

    marital status |    Freq.    Percent       Cum.
-------------------+---------------------------------
           married |    5,132      62.87      62.87
  living as couple |      654       8.01      70.88
           widowed |      189       2.32      73.20
          divorced |      397       4.86      78.06
         separated |      172       2.11      80.17
     never married |    1,619      19.83     100.00
-------------------+---------------------------------
             Total |    8,163     100.00

. tab mastat,nol

           marital |
            status |    Freq.    Percent       Cum.
-------------------+---------------------------------
                 1 |    5,132      62.87      62.87
                 2 |      654       8.01      70.88
                 3 |      189       2.32      73.20
                 4 |      397       4.86      78.06
                 5 |      172       2.11      80.17
                 6 |    1,619      19.83     100.00
-------------------+---------------------------------
             Total |    8,163     100.00
```

```
. recode mastat (6=1) (1/2=2) (4/5=3) ///
    (3=4),gen(marst2)
(7509 differences between mastat and marst2)

. lab var marst2 "marital status 4 categories"

. lab def marlab 1 "single" 2 "married" ///
    3 "sep/div" 4 "widowed"

. lab val marst2 marlab

. tab marst2

   marital |
  status 4 |
categories |      Freq.     Percent        Cum.
-----------+-----------------------------------
    single |      1,619       19.83       19.83
   married |      5,786       70.88       90.71
   sep/div |        569        6.97       97.68
   widowed |        189        2.32      100.00
-----------+-----------------------------------
     Total |      8,163      100.00
```

We now create the employment status variable:

```
ta jbstat
ta jbstat,nol
recode jbstat (1/2=1) (3=2) (7=3) (6=4) ///
    (9=4) (5=5) (8=5) (4=6) (10=.), gen(empstat)
lab var empstat "employment status"
lab def emplab 1 "employed" 2 "unemployed" ///
    3 "longterm sick" 4 "studying" ///
    5 "family care" 6 "retired"
lab val empstat emplab
ta empstat
```

```
. ta jbstat

   current labour force |
                 status |   Freq.  Percent      Cum.
------------------------+----------------------------
          self employed |     731     9.26      9.26
         in paid employ |   4,844    61.39     70.65
```

```
              unemployed |    505     6.40   77.05
                 retired |    403     5.11   82.16
             family care |    900    11.41   93.56
              ft student |    202     2.56   96.12
 long term sick/disabled |    244     3.09   99.21
         on matern leave |     13     0.16   99.38
        govt trng scheme |     22     0.28   99.66
          something else |     27     0.34  100.00
-------------------------+--------------------
                   Total | 7,891    100.00
```

```
. ta jbstat,nol

  current |
   labour |
    force |
   status |    Freq.     Percent       Cum.
----------+---------------------------------
        1 |      731        9.26        9.26
        2 |    4,844       61.39       70.65
        3 |      505        6.40       77.05
        4 |      403        5.11       82.16
        5 |      900       11.41       93.56
        6 |      202        2.56       96.12
        7 |      244        3.09       99.21
        8 |       13        0.16       99.38
        9 |       22        0.28       99.66
       10 |       27        0.34      100.00
----------+---------------------------------
    Total |    7,891      100.00
```

```
. recode jbstat (1/2=1) (3=2) (7=3) (6=4) ///
>  (9=4) (5=5) (8=5) (4=6) (10=.),gen(empstat)
(6260 differences between jbstat and empstat)

. lab var empstat "employment status"

. lab def emplab 1 "employed" 2 "unemployed" ///
>  3 "longterm sick" 4 "studying" ///
>  5 "family care" 6 "retired"

. lab val empstat emplab
```

```
. ta empstat

employment |
     status |     Freq.     Percent      Cum.
------------+----------------------------------
   employed |     5,575      70.89       70.89
 unemployed |       505       6.42       77.31
longterm sick |     244       3.10       80.42
   studying |       224       2.85       83.27
family care |       913      11.61       94.88
    retired |       403       5.12      100.00
------------+----------------------------------
      Total |     7,864     100.00
```

Next we collapse the variable for number of children into fewer categories:

su nchild
recode nchild (0=1) (1/2=2) (3/9=3), ///
   gen(numchd)
lab var numchd "children 3 categories"
lab def chdlab 1 "none" 2 "one or two" ///
   3 "three or more"
lab val numchd chdlab

```
. su nchild

Variable |     Obs       Mean   Std. Dev.   Min   Max
---------+-------------------------------------------
  nchild |    8163   .6659316   1.019895     0     9
```

```
. recode nchild (0=1) (1/2=2) (3/9=3), ///
   gen(numchd)
(6508 differences between nchild and numchd)

. lab var numchd "children 3 categories"

. lab def chdlab 1 "none" 2 "one or two" ///
   3 "three or more"

. lab val numchd chdlab

. ta numchd
```

```
   children 3 |
   categories |    Freq.    Percent      Cum.
--------------+------------------------------
        none |    5,182      63.48      63.48
  one or two |    2,443      29.93      93.41
three or more |      538       6.59     100.00
--------------+------------------------------
       Total |    8,163     100.00
```

When we have completed our recoding we produce descriptive statistics for all the variables that we will use in our future analyses.

su ghqscale d_ghq female age agecat marst2 ///
   empstat numchd

We can use the output of descriptive statistics to see if our variables have the right number of categories and cases (observations). The output below shows that some of the variables have fewer valid observations than the 8163 in our total sample. This is due to the GHQ items, employment status and marital status variables having a number of people who did not respond to the questions and so have been coded as missing values.

```
. su ghqscale d_ghq female age agecat marst2 ///
    empstat numchd

Variable |     Obs        Mean    Std. Dev.   Min   Max
---------+--------------------------------------------
ghqscale |    7714    10.76407    4.987117     0    36
   d_ghq |    7714    .1870625     .389987     0     1
  female |    8163    .5205194    .4996094     0     1
     age |    8163    39.32733    13.08993    18    65
  agecat |    8163    1.867083    .7574497     1     3
---------+--------------------------------------------
  marst2 |    8163    1.917677    .5949101     1     4
 empstat |    7864     1.93235     1.64757     1     6
  numchd |    8163    1.431092    .6140945     1     3
```

Finally, we use the **keep** command again to retain only the variables we wish to use in further analyses. The **order** command lets us order the variables in the data set if this is something you prefer. The **compress** command stores the data set in the smallest amount of space, and then the **save** command saves our new data set to our default directory for future use.

```
keep pid hid ghqscale d_ghq female age ///
    agecat marst2 empstat numchd
order pid hid ghqscale d_ghq female age ///
    agecat marst2 empstat numchd
compress
save demodata1.dta,replace
```

```
. keep pid hid ghqscale d_ghq female age ///
    agecat marst2 empstat numchd

. order pid hid ghqscale d_ghq female age ///
    agecat marst2 empstat numchd

. compress
ghqscale was float now byte

. save demodata1.dta,replace
(note: file demodata1.dta not found)
file demodata1.dta saved
```

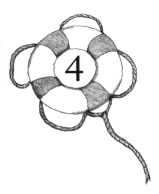

4 Manipulating data

SORTING DATA

Often you need to sort data; that is, to organize the cases or rows according to the categories of one or more variables. There are a number of reasons for wanting to do this, the main ones being: (1) preparing data to be merged with other data sets (more on that later); and (2) if you want to produce statistics separately for different groups – men and women or different countries, for example.

To sort your data, type **sort** followed by the variable or variables you want to sort by. If you want to sort by sex:

```
sort sex
```

The command will sort the data by the categories of the variable *sex* from the lowest to the highest. Now if you want to know the descriptive statistics of some variables by *sex*, you can examine them by using the prefix command **by**. A colon (:) must follow the variable or variables by which you sorted (and by which you want to have your output organized). For example, if you wanted the mean age for men and women you would use the command:

```
by sex: su age
```

If you have not sorted your data and try to use the **by** command then Stata will return the error message (in red): not sorted.

There is more detail on the command **su** to produce descriptive data and alternative commands in Chapter 5.

In the latest versions of Stata, the **by** and **sort** prefix commands can be combined into one prefix command, **bysort**, which can be used when organizing results by groups. For the same example of the mean ages of men and women you could use

bysort sex:su age

As with the **by** command, it is necessary to place a colon (:) after
the variable(s) to sort on.

```
. bysort sex:su age

-----------------------------------------------------------
-> sex = male

    Variable |      Obs        Mean   Std. Dev.   Min    Max
-------------+---------------------------------------------
         age |     4833    43.37099    17.98608    16     94

-----------------------------------------------------------
-> sex = female

    Variable |      Obs        Mean   Std. Dev.   Min    Max
-------------+---------------------------------------------
         age |     5431     45.5511    18.82718    16     97
```

The **bysort** command can also be used with as many variables as you need to create the subgroups you are interested in.
The **bysort** variable(s) should generally refer to a categorical
variable or variables. For example, if you were interested in
extending the previous example and wanted to know the mean
ages of men and women but further broken down by their marital
status you would use

bysort sex mastat: su age

The order of the two variables after **bysort** determines how the
output is presented. The above command produces the (partial)
results shown below with the mean ages of men by their marital
status; this would be followed by the mean ages of women by their
marital status. This is because in the variable *sex*, men are coded 1
and women coded 2.

```
. bysort sex mastat:su age

-----------------------------------------------------------
-> sex = male, mastat = married

    Variable |      Obs        Mean   Std. Dev.   Min    Max
-------------+---------------------------------------------
         age |     2947    48.60333    15.08131    18     94
```

```
-----------------------------------------------------
-> sex = male, mastat = living a

   Variable |    Obs        Mean  Std. Dev.  Min   Max
------------+----------------------------------------
        age |    334   33.45808   12.36032    17    91


-----------------------------------------------------
-> sex = male, mastat = widowed

   Variable |    Obs        Mean  Std. Dev.  Min   Max
------------+----------------------------------------
        age |    169   73.70414   10.53543    35    91


-----------------------------------------------------
-> sex = male, mastat = divorced

   Variable |    Obs        Mean  Std. Dev.  Min   Max
------------+----------------------------------------
        age |    150   47.88667   12.97056    23    82

etc
```

If you wanted to organize your results so that you could more easily compare the mean ages of men and women within each category of marital status, then you may find it better to use

bysort mastat sex: su age

This produces the (partial) results shown below where you can see that the mean ages for both men and women are shown for those who are married, cohabiting, etc.

```
. bysort mastat sex :su age

-----------------------------------------------------
-> mastat = married, sex = male
   Variable |    Obs        Mean  Std. Dev.  Min   Max
------------+----------------------------------------
        age |   2947   48.60333   15.08131    18    94


-----------------------------------------------------
-> mastat = married, sex = female
   Variable |    Obs        Mean  Std. Dev.  Min   Max
------------+----------------------------------------
        age |   3062   45.84651   14.68746    18    89

etc
```

The command after **bysort mastat sex:** could be a range of operations that we haven't covered yet. It is possible to have separate estimations for groups you have specified using many statistical functions, such as correlations, regressions, and *t*-tests, just to name a few. But it is worth noting that using the **bysort** command does mean some restrictions on other commands you can use.

MERGING AND APPENDING DATA

There may be times when you will want to join two or more data files with one another. There are two main ways – merging and appending. Figure 4.1 illustrates the basic difference between them. Merging adds one file horizontally to the right of another file in the spreadsheet, and appending adds one file vertically to the bottom of another file. The data file that is already open in Stata is referred to as the *master* data and the data file to be added is referred to as the *using* data. In both the **merge** and **append** commands you will specify the data to be added by **using data.dta** part of the command.

For example, you might need to merge your data files if you have follow-up data on the same set of respondents, and this would add more variables to the rows containing the master data. If your study was collecting data from two or more locations where the data are entered then you might need to append all the data files together into one large data file.

Merging data

The **merge** command is best illustrated with an example. Here, we have a small data file from 2004 (called 2004data.dta) that contains information on five people's age (*age04*), income in units of 10,000 (*inc04*) and marital status (*mstat04*); each person has an identifying number (*id*).

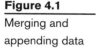

Figure 4.1
Merging and
appending data

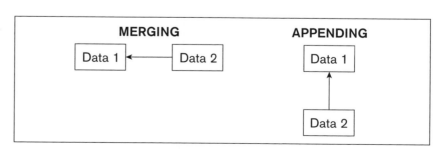

id	age04	inc04	mstat04
1	25	55	married
2	24	66	single
3	23	45	divorced
4	24	27	married
5	32	100	cohabiting

You have data on age, income and marital status from the same five people in 2005 (called 2005data.dta) and want to merge these data with the 2004 data.

id	age05	inc05	mstat05
1	26	57	married
2	25	78	single
3	24	32	divorced
4	25	59	divorced
5	33	200	married

You would end up with a file that was organized like this:

id	age04	inc04	mstat04	age05	inc05	mstat05
1	25	55	married	26	57	married
2	24	66	single	25	78	single
3	23	45	divorced	24	32	divorced
4	24	27	married	25	59	divorced
5	32	100	cohabiting	33	200	married

The data from the year 2005 is added to the right of the 2004 data for all cases. Another thing to note when you merge files is the naming of the variables. If the variables in both the 2004 and 2005 data had simply been called *age*, *inc* and *mstat*, then when you attempted to merge them Stata would not return an error message but use the values for the variable from the master data! So you must ensure that your variables have unique names before you merge data files.

To do this step-by-step proceed as follows:

1. Make sure both data files are sorted on the variable you wish to merge by – in this example, the *id* variable is used as it is common to both data files. If you regularly merge data then we recommend that you get into the habit of sorting on the merge variable before you save your data. This way you know the data is sorted and then can omit the first stage of the do file example below.
2. Open the data file that is to be the master data – in this case the 2004 data.
3. Merge the 2005 data on to the 2004 data.
4. Save the new data file under a new name.

The do file to do this would look like this:

```
cd datafolder                /* set default folder */

use 2005data,clear           /* open 2005 data */
sort id                      /* sort by id ready
                                to merge */
save 2005data,replace        /* save sorted 2005
                                data */

use 2004data,clear           /* open 2004 data */
sort id                      /* sort by id ready
                                to merge */

merge id using 2005data      /* merge on 2005 data
                                by id */

sort id                      /* ensure sorted by
                                id */
save newdata,replace         /* save as new file */
```

Alternatively, you can use the **sort** option in the **merge** command which means the do file would be:

```
cd datafolder
use 2004data,clear
merge id using 2005data,sort
save newdata,replace
```

Rarely is real-world data as straightforward as the above example, and it is more than likely that any follow-up data will have respondents who have dropped out of the study. To add a further twist, it is also possible that new people have entered the study. This is the case in many of the household-based surveys when a child reaches a certain age to be included in the study. Stata produces a variable called _merge that will help you determine how many cases have dropped out, entered or remained in the data.

To extend the previous example, suppose you now have two sets of data – one from 2001 and one from 2002 – with the same variables as before, but not all of the people are in both years. The 2001 data are:

id	age01	inc01	mstat01
1	35	45	married
2	24	66	single
3	28	25	divorced
4	24	27	married
5	32	100	cohabiting
6	42	35	married
7	26	14	single
8	38	23	married
9	40	85	cohabiting
10	44	27	divorced

The 2002 data are:

id	age02	inc02	mstat02
1	36	57	married
3	29	32	divorced
4	25	59	divorced
5	33	200	married
7	27	14	single
8	39	23	married
9	41	85	cohabiting
11	18	10	single
12	21	15	single

If you merged these two files you would end up with a file that was organized like this:

id	age01	inc01	mstat01	age02	inc02	mstat02
1	35	45	married	36	57	married
2	24	66	single	.	.	.
3	28	25	divorced	29	32	divorced
4	24	27	married	25	25	divorced
5	32	100	cohabiting	33	120	married
6	42	35	married	.	.	.
7	26	14	single	27	14	single
8	38	23	married	39	24	married
9	40	85	cohabiting	41	80	cohabiting
10	44	27	divorced	.	.	.
11	.	.	.	18	10	single
12	.	.	.	21	15	single

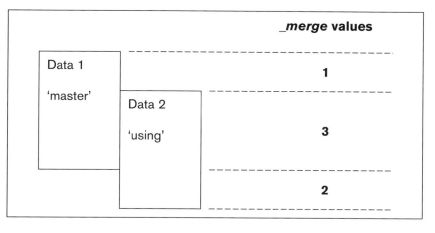

Figure 4.2
The _merge
variable

In this case, you can make use of the new variable _merge which will have been created and placed at the end of your data file after merging the two data files – the bottom of your list of variables. The variable _merge is very important. It gives you information on the success of your merge. There are three codes associated with _merge (see Figure 4.2):

_merge = 1, observations/cases from your master data;
_merge = 2, observations/cases from your using data;
_merge = 3, observations/cases from both your master and using
    data.

You should be very careful with merges that do not equal 3. Those coded 1 in this case refer to cases lost from 2001 to 2002, while those coded 2 refer to cases that appear only in 2002 and not in 2001. Merges that equal 3 mean that the observation/case was present in both years.

The do file for this merge would look like this:

```
cd datafolder              /* set default folder */

use 2001data,clear         /* open 2001 data */
merge id using 2002data,sort   /* merge on 2002
                                  data by id */

ta _merge                  /* inspect _merge
                              variable */

drop _merge                /* drop _merge not
                              needed? */

sort id                    /* ensure sorted by id */
save newdata,replace       /* save as new file */
```

If you run the above do file, part of your results should look like this:

```
. ta _merge

    _merge |    Freq.    percent        Cum.
-----------+-----------------------------------
         1 |         3      25.00       25.00
         2 |         2      16.67       41.67
         3 |         7      58.33      100.00
-----------+-----------------------------------
     Total |        12     100.00
```

Seven cases were in both the master and using data (_merge = 3), 3 cases were in the master data only (_merge = 1), and 2 cases were in the using data only (_merge = 2). We recommend that you tabulate the _merge variable to check your merges, especially when you first attempt this type of data manipulation. The **merge** command has a number of options that allow you to keep only the cases for some of the _merge values, but to start with you should view the tabulated results and then decide if you wish to delete any of the cases. Remember to drop the _merge variable if it is no longer needed or rename it if you need to keep it but have other merges to perform, because if you don't Stata will return an error saying that the _merge variable already exists.

In these simple examples we have only used one variable (*id*) to uniquely identify cases in both data sets, but the **merge** command can specify more than one variable if a combination of variables is what uniquely identifies each case (which is often the case in large-scale data sets). For example:

merge id_1 id_2 id_3 using otherdata,sort

Using the **sort** option in this way implies that the matching variables (*id_1*, *id_2* and *id_3*) uniquely identify the same cases in both data sets. There are other options to the **merge** command when this situation doesn't apply, but these are quite advanced techniques.

Merging data files of different levels (hierarchical data structures)

Merging files of different levels is quite common when, for example, you have data from individuals (in an individual level data file) and data from the households in which the individuals live (in a household level file). Another example would be an individual level data file on people's experiences of and attitudes to crime and data at neighbourhood level on crime rates and police efficiency. Again, this process is best illustrated with an example. In this one you have an individual level data file (each row is data from a person) and a household level data file (each row refers to data about the household).

In the individual level file (individual.dta), there is a person identifier (*id*) which uniquely identifies each individual and a household identifier (*hid*) which uniquely identifies each household; as you can see, most households have more than one person. In these data, three people live in household 1, two people in household 2, one person in household 3, one person in household 4, and three people in household 5.

id	hid	age	inc	mstat
1	1	25	55	married
2	1	24	66	single
3	1	23	45	divorced
4	2	24	27	married
5	2	32	100	married
6	3	54	78	single
7	4	33	0	single
8	5	21	74	single
9	5	33	0	single
10	5	21	77	single

The household level file (household.dta) has information on household size and region of the country. The variable that is common to the individual level file and the household level file is *hid*. In order to match data from the household level file onto the

individual level file, you would need to make sure that a common
identifier is present in each file type.

hid	hhsize	region
1	3	south
2	2	north
3	1	east
4	1	west
5	3	north

When you merge these files by their common identifier (*hid*) you
will end up with a file that has the household characteristics
merged on to each individual:

id	hid	age	inc	mstat	hhsize	region
1	1	25	55	married	3	south
2	1	24	66	single	3	south
3	1	23	45	divorced	3	south
4	2	24	27	married	2	north
5	2	32	100	married	2	north
6	3	54	78	single	1	east
7	4	33	0	single	1	west
8	5	21	74	single	3	north
9	5	33	0	single	3	north
10	5	21	77	single	3	north

The do file for this merge would look similar to the one for
merging the individual data files, but this time sorting on *hid* as it
is the common variable to merge on.

To have Stata merge on multiple rows of the master data, the commands **merge** or **joinby** can be used. Both commands tell Stata to match on all possible pairs between the master and using data on the common variable(s) (in this case *hid*) and give pretty much the same results. The **joinby** command, however, does not automatically generate the _merge variable as with the **merge** command. This is because Stata only matches the possible rows of data. If you specify the option **unmatched(both)** (shortened to **unm(b)** below) to the **joinby** command then a _merge variable is generated with the same features as with the **merge** command. There are a number of other options to the **joinby** command for more complex matching situations.

```
cd datafolder                        /*set default folder*/

use household,clear                  /*open household
                                        data*/
sort hid                             /*sort by hid*/
save household,replace               /*save sorted data*/

use individual,clear                 /*open individual
                                        data*/
sort hid                             /*sort by hid for
                                        merge*/
joinby hid using household,unm(b)    /*join hhold
                                               data by hid*/

ta _merge                            /*inspect _merge*/
drop _merge                          /*drop _merge*/

sort hid id                          /*sort by hid and id*/
save newdata,replace                 /*save as new file*/
```

In this example, all cases will have a value of 3 on the _merge variable, but often that is not the case in real-world data. Some respondents may have provided individual data but not household data. In this case, they would be _merge = 1 as they are in the master data (the individual level file) but not in the using file (the household level file). Conversely, if there is household data but no matching individual level data then these households would be _merge = 2 as they are in the using data but not in the master data.

For merging housing and individual data using the **merge** command, see the demonstration exercise later in this chapter.

Appending data

The **append** command is also best illustrated with an example. In this example you have collected a small set of data from town A (called townAdata.dta) and another researcher has collected similar data from town B (called townBdata.dta). Both sets of data contain information on five people's year of birth (*yob*), employment status (*empstat*) and income in units of 10,000 (*inc*), and each person has an identifying number (*id*). Here are the town A data:

id	yob	empstat	inc
101	1968	employed	45
102	1973	not working	66
103	1974	employed	45
104	1980	student	14
105	1963	employed	80

Here are the town B data:

id	yob	empstat	inc
201	1977	employed	57
202	1960	employed	78
203	1982	not working	32
204	1975	not working	59
205	1968	employed	91

There are three issues to deal with before you can append these data.

1. You need to make sure that the person identifier variable (*id*) has different values in both sets of data. It would have been easy for both data collectors to use the numbers 1 to 5. In

this example, the people in town A have identifiers 101 to 105 and those in town B have 201 to 205.

2. You need to make sure that the variable names are identical in both sets of data, otherwise Stata will treat them as different variables and put the data in different columns (see Box 4.1).

3. You should consider adding a new variable to each set of data that indicates what town the people come from. In each set of data this technically will not be a variable as the values are constant for all people in the data, but after the data files are appended it will vary depending on which town the people are from.

Box 4.1: Variable names when appending data

If the variable names, for the same variable, are different in the data sets then Stata treats them as different variables and puts them in different columns. For example, if income is called *inc* in the town A data and *income* in town B data, then after you append the data it will look like this:

id	yob	empstat	inc	income	town
101	1968	employed	45	.	1
102	1973	not working	66	.	1
103	1974	employed	45	.	1
104	1980	student	14	.	1
105	1963	employed	80	.	1
201	1977	employed	.	57	2
202	1960	employed	.	78	2
203	1982	not working	.	32	2
204	1975	not working	.	59	2
205	1968	employed	.	91	2

After you create a new variable for the town (where 1 = town A and 2 = town B) and append the sets of data you end up with a file like this:

id	yob	empstat	inc	town
101	1968	employed	45	1
102	1973	not working	66	1
103	1974	employed	45	1
104	1980	student	14	1
105	1963	employed	80	1
201	1977	employed	57	2
202	1960	employed	78	2
203	1982	not working	32	2
204	1975	not working	59	2
205	1968	employed	91	2

The do file to append these sets of data would look like:

```
cd datafolder                /* set default
                                folder */

use townBdata,clear          /* open town B data */
gen town=2                   /* new variable
                                town */
save townBdata,replace       /* save data */
use townAdata,clear          /* open individual
                                data */
gen town=1                   /* new variable
                                town */
append using townBdata       /* append town B
                                data */

sort id                      /* ensure sorted
                                by id */
save newdata,replace         /* save as new file */
```

LONGITUDINAL DATA

Longitudinal data comes from surveys or studies that have collected information from the same source on more that one occasion. This type of data is also regularly referred to in the social sciences as 'panel' data because the data is observational rather than experimental. The definitions of 'longitudinal' and 'panel' data are often blurred at the edges and sometimes the terms are used interchangeably as the surveys tend to be more complex than a simple panel. For a fuller discussion on types of longitudinal data, see Frees (2004), Singer and Willett (2003) and Wooldridge (2002).

One important concept to emphasize, before we tackle data manipulation, is the difference between balanced and unbalanced panel data. In a balanced panel, there are data at all points of time for all individuals (or other source of data) in the panel. In an unbalanced panel, the number of individuals at each point of time may change as some drop out or some new people enter the study. We have illustrated this in Figure 4.3. In the top half of the figure we show a balanced panel of five people who are present at all three data collection points. In the lower half we show an unbalanced panel that starts with five people at the first time point. By the time of the second data collection there are four left in the

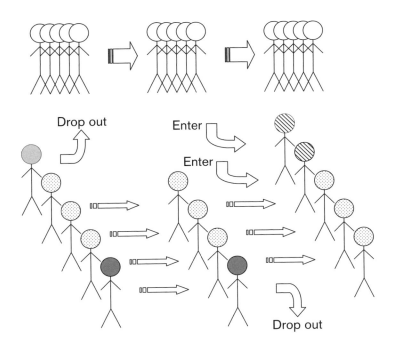

Figure 4.3

Balanced and unbalanced panels

panel with one person (shaded light grey) dropping out of the study. At the third data collection, there are again five people in the study but only three are original members (dotted) as one more person (shaded dark grey) has dropped out but two new people (stripes) have joined the study.

Most large longitudinal studies have fairly complex rules about who stays in, leaves or enters the study as time goes on. These are sometimes known as 'following rules' and need to be thoroughly understood before using the data for any project. As a general rule, panel studies based on families or households have more complex following rules than those based on a cohort with some common characteristic, such as a birth cohort that are born in the same week. The dynamics of modern family life – partnering, marriage, births, deaths, separation and divorce – naturally require more complex following rules than a tightly defined cohort of individuals. However, even what may appear to be straightforward cohort studies have developed into far more complex studies.

Longitudinal data may come from a variety of data sources. We often see graphs or charts of a country's economic indicators such as gross national product, unemployment or public spending for a number of years to show a trend over time. These are longitudinal data, and a data set could very well contain similar information from a number of countries. Similarly, within a given country, data over time could be collected from county or state level, hospitals, schools or police forces.

Longitudinal data need some consideration to enable them to be used for analysis. This primarily rests with the structure of the data required by Stata. For many types of analysis, Stata requires the data to be in unit/time format (although some types of analysis can be done in wide format). Unit is the source of the data – person, country, etc. – and time is the interval between data collection. So, for example, for the individual data from the British Household Panel Survey (collected yearly) the data format would be person/year and for monthly country level data it would be country/month format. In the first example, each row in the data spreadsheet would contain data from one person for one year of data collection. Therefore, each person has as many rows of data as the number of years they have been in the survey.

In the example data below there are four people, with $id =$ 001, 002, 003 and 004. Person 001 has three years' worth of data, which can be seen from the identifier appearing in three rows of data, and the time variable (*year*) shows that these data are for 2001, 2002 and 2003. Person 002 has only one year's data, for 2002. Person 003 has five years' data, but with data missing for 2002. Person 004 has three years' data, but not from consecutive years.

id	year	age	mstat
001	2001	16	single
001	2002	17	single
001	2003	18	single
002	2002	67	widowed
003	1999	27	single
003	2000	28	married
003	2001	29	married
003	2003	31	separated
003	2004	32	separated
004	1999	44	married
004	2002	47	married
004	2004	49	divorced

One important thing to note when your data are organized in person/year (or more generally unit/time) format is that the *id* number does not uniquely identify a particular row of data. It is the combination of the *id* and the *year* variable that is unique to each row of data.

When your data are arranged in person/year format it is possible to easily see the changes to other variables over time. In the above example, you can see that person 001 is 16 years old in 2001 and is single. They stay in the study for two more years, 2002 and 2003, as they age to 17 and 18 years old and they stay single at all three time points. It is worth noting here that in real survey data the age variable may not increase as uniformly as we have shown here, as survey dates may differ from year to year. Person 003 stays in the study for five time points from 1999 to 2004, but data from 2002 is missing. In that time they age from 27 to 32 and their marital status (*mstat*) shows that they married between the 1999 and 2000 interviews, then separated between the 2001 and 2003 interviews.

Stata has a number of features that make it easy to manipulate longitudinal data and to gain insights into your data structure. Here, we demonstrate some of the basic features you may need to start getting a handle on manipulating longitudinal data. Stata contains many more complex features for use with longitudinal data which can be employed when you are comfortable with the basic techniques. More details on these advanced techniques can be found in Rabe-Hesketh and Skrondal (2008).

_n AND _N

These two features are commonly used in conjunction with a **generate** command to give you some information about the structure of your data. They will help you answer questions such as 'How many people are in the study at all time points?' and 'What is the distribution of the number of times people are in the study?'

To start, the data from each time point need to be appended to each other with a time variable specified similar to that described earlier in the chapter with the example for the town A and town B data, but instead of generating the *town* variable you need to generate a time variable. To illustrate the use of **_n** and **_N** we will continue with the example data described immediately above. Before the **_n** and **_N** features are used to generate new variables, the data must be sorted on the *id* and *year* variables.

We then use the **generate** command and the **_n** and **_N** features to make two new variables (*seq* and *tot*) in the data:

```
sort id year
by id: gen seq = _n
by id: gen tot = _N
```

These commands would produce the following results:

id	year	age	mstat	seq	tot
001	2001	16	single	1	3
001	2002	17	single	2	3
001	2003	18	single	3	3
002	2002	67	widowed	1	1
003	1999	27	single	1	5
003	2000	28	married	2	5
003	2001	29	married	3	5
003	2003	31	separated	4	5
003	2004	32	separated	5	5
004	1999	44	married	1	3
004	2002	47	married	2	3
004	2004	49	divorced	3	3

Using combinations of the *year*, *seq* and *tot* variables, you can find out some core information about your data. For example, from the above small data set, you can **tabulate** the *year* variable conditional on the *seq* variable equalling 1 and you will get the number of people by their first year in the study.

```
ta year if seq==1

. ta year if seq==1
       year |      Freq.     Percent        Cum.
------------+-----------------------------------
       1999 |          2       50.00       50.00
       2001 |          1       25.00       75.00
       2002 |          1       25.00      100.00
------------+-----------------------------------
      Total |          4      100.00
```

This shows that two people were first observed in 1999 then one each in 2001 and 2002. Other combinations can tell you the distribution of the individuals' number of years in the study:

ta tot if seq==1

```
. ta tot if seq==1

       tot |      Freq.     Percent        Cum.
-----------+-----------------------------------
         1 |          1       25.00       25.00
         3 |          2       50.00       75.00
         5 |          1       25.00      100.00
-----------+-----------------------------------
     Total |          4      100.00
```

This shows that one person was in the study at only one time point, two people were observed three times and one person was observed five times.

The following command identifies the last year in the study for each person:

ta year if seq==tot

```
. ta year if seq==tot

      year |      Freq.     Percent        Cum.
-----------+-----------------------------------
      2002 |          1       25.00       25.00
      2003 |          1       25.00       50.00
      2004 |          2       50.00      100.00
-----------+-----------------------------------
     Total |          4      100.00
```

The last year in the study for each person is identified when *seq* = *tot*, so this tells you that one person was last observed in 2002, another in 2003 and the other two people last observed in 2004.

While all this information is useful, none of it tells us what years the people were in the study between their first and last observation. There is a potential maximum of six observations in these data as the earliest date is 1999 and the latest is 2004, but no one was observed six times. One person (*id* 003) was observed five times, but is missing for 2002. There are ways of using the *year*

Box 4.2: Long and wide files

Longitudinal data or data with repeated measures need to be organized in a way that allows Stata to compute the appropriate tests some of which we cover in Chapter 7. The most common way of referring to the two main types of data organization is as 'long' and 'wide' files.

Long files are where the data are 'stacked', usually constructed by using the **append** command. In this way each row contains data from a person at a particular time point. In panel data this could mean each row represents a person/year but in data from a pre- and post-test experiment each row would represent a person/test. Then the number of rows for each person matches the number of times they have been interviewed or tested.

Wide files are where each row contains all the variables for that person. For example, the data may be a set of variables collected in 2002 then to the right of them would be variables from 2003 and so on. So each person has a row and the number of variables depends on the number of times interviewed or tested. Wide files are usually constructed using the **merge** command.

variable in conjunction with the _**n** and _**N** functions to identify these breaks in observations as Stata can look within the rows with the same *id* value to see if numbers are sequential or not.

However, these techniques are beyond the scope of this book and we just want to draw your attention to them and to some other capabilities that you may want to progress on to. The comparative ease of handling longitudinal data is one of the main reasons why many people change to using Stata. If you too take the route to longitudinal data analysis then there are many books available; we would also suggest taking a course as some of the issues are best worked out in the classroom as they can take a little time to get your head around.

MORE ADVANCED DATA HANDLING

Two other more advanced data handling commands to be aware of are **reshape** and **expand**. These are both very powerful commands. Very briefly, **reshape** allows you to change data from wide to long format and vice versa. The most common use is to change wide files into long files as Stata has far more capability using long files. You need to invest some time in ensuring the data and variables are correctly formatted, because then the command is rather simple.

For example, we have a small data set as seen in the Data Editor:

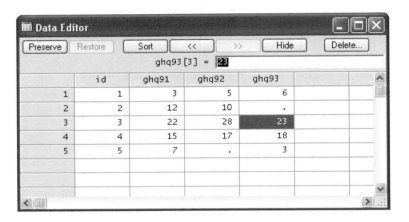

There is the *id* variable and then three variables *ghq91*, *ghq92* and *ghq93*. This is the format of the variable names that Stata needs to perform the **reshape** command; a common prefix and a numeric suffix. Stata will interpret this as the same measure (*ghq*) taken at times 91, 92 and 93. Then we use the **reshape** command and specify we want these data changed to long format. After **long** we put the common variable prefix, *ghq*, then after the comma tell Stata that the identifier variable is *id*.

reshape long ghq,i(id)

```
. reshape long ghq,i(id)
(note: j = 91 92 93)

Data                                    wide  ->  long
-----------------------------------------------------
Number of obs.                             5  ->    15
Number of variables                        4  ->     3
j variable (3 values)                         ->    _j
xij variables:
                        ghq91 ghq92 ghq93  ->   ghq
```

The output tells us that the number of observations has changed from 5 to 15: five people observed three times each, even taking into account missing values. The number of variables has changed from 4 to 3: *id*, *ghq* and a new variable *_j*. It also tells us that *_j* has three values. This is the 'time' variable, and we expect this to be 91, 92 and 93. If we look in the Data Browser we see the following:

	id	_j	ghq	
1	1	91	3	
2	1	92	5	
3	1	93	6	
4	2	91	12	
5	2	92	10	
6	2	93	.	
7	3	91	22	
8	3	92	28	
9	3	93	23	
10	4	91	15	
11	4	92	17	
12	4	93	18	
13	5	91	7	
14	5	92	.	
15	5	93	3	

Obviously these reshaping techniques can get very complicated, but at this stage we would just like you to be aware of some of Stata's capabilities. Compare **reshape** with the **xpose** command that we mention in Chapter 7.

The other command is **expand**. This command tells Stata to add rows of data for each case so that there are as many rows for each case as in the specified variable. The specified variable is usually a time variable so that after the expansion each row represents a time point. In this simple example we use a variable *years*. The first case (*id*=1) has a value of 3 in years, so after the expansion there will be three rows of data. If the value of *years* was 1, less than 1 or missing then only the original single row of data would remain.

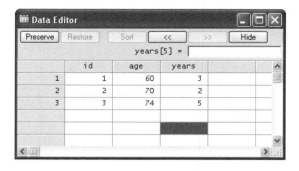

The expansion is done by:

```
expand years
sort id
```

```
. expand years
(7 observations created)
```

Now the data look like this:

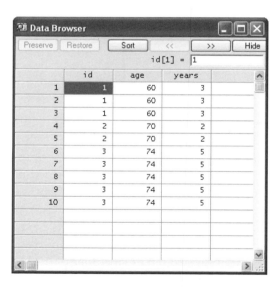

You can see that each case now has the same number of rows as the value of the *years* variable. You could now use this to change the age at each observation to match the one-year increase in time by using:

```
bysort id: gen seq=_n-1
replace age=age+seq
```

Now the data look like this:

	id	age	years	seq
1	1	60	3	0
2	1	61	3	1
3	1	62	3	2
4	2	70	2	0
5	2	71	2	1
6	3	74	5	0
7	3	75	5	1
8	3	76	5	2
9	3	77	5	3
10	3	78	5	4

We used the **_n** function to make a new variable *seq* but instead of starting at 1 we used **_n-1** so the count started at 0 for each id. Then we replaced the old values for *age* with new values of *age* plus the *seq* value. Again, this is just a very brief indication of the data manipulation capabilities of Stata.

DEMONSTRATION EXERCISE

In Chapter 3 we manipulated the individual level variables and saved a new data set called demodata1.dta. In this part of the exercise we merge the individual data file with household level data in the hhexampledata.dta data set to add the region of country variable.

First, we need to ensure that the household level data set is correctly sorted ready for the merge as we are using a step-by-step approach rather than the **sort** option in the **merge** command. The data are opened and then inspected.

```
use hhexampledata.dta, clear
keep hid region
su hid
```

```
. su hid

Variable |      Obs      Mean   Std. Dev.        Min        Max
---------+-----------------------------------------------------
     hid |     5511   1396155    219476.6    1000209    1761811
```

From this output you can see that in the hhexampledata.dta file there are data on 5511 households as each has its own unique identifier (*hid*).

Next we examine the *region* variable prior to collapsing the categories into the ones we want to use in our analyses.

ta region
ta region, nol

```
. tab region

      region / metropolitan |
                       area |   Freq.   Percent     Cum.
--------------------------+------------------------------
             inner london |     247      4.48      4.48
             outer london |     348      6.31     10.80
          r. of south east |     990     17.96     28.76
               south west |     493      8.95     37.71
              east anglia |     208      3.77     41.48
            east midlands |     399      7.24     48.72
west midlands conurbation |     240      4.35     53.08
       r. of west midlands |     263      4.77     57.85
        greater manchester |     242      4.39     62.24
               merseyside |     131      2.38     64.62
          r. of north west |     247      4.48     69.10
          south yorkshire |     151      2.74     71.84
           west yorkshire |     205      3.72     75.56
   r. of yorks & humberside |     175      3.18     78.73
              tyne & wear |     144      2.61     81.35
             r. of north |     216      3.92     85.27
                    wales |     281      5.10     90.36
                 scotland |     531      9.64    100.00
--------------------------+------------------------------
                    Total |   5,511    100.00
```

```
. tab region,nol

   region / |
metropolita |
    n area  |     Freq.     Percent        Cum.
------------+---------------------------------
         1  |      247        4.48        4.48
         2  |      348        6.31       10.80
         3  |      990       17.96       28.76
         4  |      493        8.95       37.71
         5  |      208        3.77       41.48
         6  |      399        7.24       48.72
         7  |      240        4.35       53.08
         8  |      263        4.77       57.85
         9  |      242        4.39       62.24
        10  |      131        2.38       64.62
        11  |      247        4.48       69.10
        12  |      151        2.74       71.84
        13  |      205        3.72       75.56
        14  |      175        3.18       78.73
        15  |      144        2.61       81.35
        16  |      216        3.92       85.27
        17  |      281        5.10       90.36
        18  |      531        9.64      100.00
------------+---------------------------------
     Total  |    5,511      100.00
```

As you can see from the output, there are 18 categories in the *region* variable. We recode this variable into a new variable (*region2*) which has seven categories: London, South, Midlands, Northwest, North and Northeast, Wales, and Scotland.

```
recode region (1/2=1) (3/5=2) (6/7=3) ///
   (9/11=4) (12/16=5) (17=6) (18=7), ///
   gen(region2)
lab var region2 "regions 7 categories"
lab def region 1 "London" 2 "South" ///
   3 "Midlands" 4 "Northwest" 5 "North and ///
   Northeast" 6 "Wales" 7 "Scotland"
lab val region2 region
tab region2
```

```
. tab region2
         regions 7 |
        categories |      Freq.      Percent        Cum.
-------------------+-----------------------------------
            London |        595        10.80        10.80
             South |      1,691        30.68        41.48
          Midlands |        902        16.37        57.85
         Northwest |        620        11.25        69.10
North and Northeast |       891        16.17        85.27
             Wales |        281         5.10        90.36
          Scotland |        531         9.64       100.00
-------------------+-----------------------------------
             Total |      5,511       100.00
```

The two variables *hid* and *region2* are kept then sorted on the *hid* (household identifier) variable and then saved with a new file name.

keep hid region2
sort hid
save hhdata1, replace

Next, we open the individual level data set saved from Chapter 3 (demodata1.dta) and sort by the matching variable (*hid*) before merging the household level data.

use demodata1, clear
sort hid
merge hid using hhdata1
ta _merge

```
. merge hid using hhdata1.dta
variable hid does not uniquely identify
observations in the master data

. ta _merge
     _merge |      Freq.      Percent        Cum.
------------+-----------------------------------
          2 |      1,092        11.80        11.80
          3 |      8,163        88.20       100.00
------------+-----------------------------------
      Total |      9,255       100.00
```

Stata gives a warning that the *hid* variable does not uniquely identify cases in the master (individual) data. We would expect this because individuals in the same household will have the same *hid* value. The **merge** command creates a new variable *_merge* in the data. To inspect the cases involved in the merge process we tabulate the *_merge* variable (see Figure 4.2). From this output you can see that none of the cases were only in the master data (the individual level file) as there is no value 1 in the *_merge* variable. *_merge=2* indicates how many cases were only in the using data file, which means there were no cases in the individual file to match onto. This is to be expected as we dropped cases from the individual file as we are only concerned with working age respondents. *_merge=3* indicates that there were 8163 cases in both the master and using files. This corresponds to the number of individuals in the demodata1.dta file – see the output from this demonstration exercise in Chapter 3 or summarize the *pid* variable to check.

```
. su pid

Variable |    Obs       Mean   Std. Dev.        Min        Max
---------+-------------------------------------------------------
     pid |   8163   1.47e+07    2640230   1.00e+07   1.91e+07
```

Now we only want to keep the 8163 individual cases with matched household data and then we have no more use for the *_merge* variable so we drop it from the data set.

keep if _merge==3
drop _merge

Check the new data set before saving under a new name

su _all
compress
save demodata2.dta, replace

```
. su _all

    Variable |       Obs        Mean    Std. Dev.         Min         Max
-------------+--------------------------------------------------------------
         pid |      8163     1.47e+07     2640230    1.00e+07    1.91e+07
         hid |      8163     1393652     220058.3     1000381     1761811
     ghqscale |      7714    10.76407    4.987117           0          36
        d_ghq |      7714    .1870625     .389987           0           1
       female |      8163    .5205194    .4996094           0           1
-------------+--------------------------------------------------------------
         age |      8163    39.32733    13.08993          18          65
      agecat |      8163    1.867083    .7574497           1           3
      marst2 |      8163    1.917677    .5949101           1           4
     empstat |      7864     1.93235     1.64757           1           6
      numchd |      8163    1.431092    .6140945           1           3
-------------+--------------------------------------------------------------
     region2 |      8163    3.435869    1.816138           1           7

. compress

. save demodata2.dta, replace
(note: file demodata2.dta not found)
file demodata2.dta saved
```

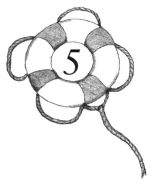

Descriptive Statistics and Graphs

5

In this chapter we look at how Stata produces descriptive, or uni-variate, statistics. These techniques are commonly used to explore the data before making decisions about further analysis and, when reporting analyses, to give the reader information about the nature and categories of the variables that have been used.

Deciding which statistics to use to describe a variable largely depends on the level of measurement of the variable. Here we refer to nominal, ordinal and interval levels of measurement. More details are given in Box 5.1 if you need them.

Box 5.1: A refresher on levels of measurement

Level of measurement is one of the fundamental building blocks in quantitative data analysis. Almost every statistical process starts with recognizing the level of measurement of the variable(s) to be used. It is vital that level of measurement is thoroughly understood.

Nominal

At the *nominal* level of measurement, numbers or other symbols are assigned to a set of categories for the purpose of naming, labelling or classifying the observations. Gender is an example of a nominal level variable. Using the numbers 1 and 2, for instance, we can classify our observations into the categories 'female' and 'male', with 1 representing female and 2 representing male. We could use any of a variety of words to represent the different cate-gories of a nominal variable; however, when numbers are used to represent the different categories, we do not imply anything about the magnitude or quantitative difference between the categories.

▶

▶ Other examples of nominal level variables are: ethnicity, nationality, race and case/control.

Ordinal

Ordinal level variables assign numbers to rank-ordered categories ranging from lowest to highest. The classic ordinal level measure is a Likert scale that has categories of strongly disagree, disagree, neither agree or disagree, agree, and strongly agree. We can say that a person in the category 'strongly agree' agrees with the statement more than a person in the 'agree' category, but we do not know the magnitude of the differences between the categories; that is, we don't know how much more agreement there is when 'strongly agree' is compared to 'agree'. Another example of an ordinal level variable is age groups such as young, middle-age and old or even 16–40, 41–64, 65 and over.

Interval/ratio

For *interval/ratio* (usually just referred to as interval) level of measurement the categories (or values) of a variable can be rank-ordered *and* the differences between these categories (or values) are constant. Examples of variables measured at the interval/ratio level are age, income, height and weight. With all these variables we can compare values not only in terms of which is larger or smaller, but also in terms of how much larger or smaller one is compared with another. In some discussions of levels of measurement you will see a distinction made between interval/ratio variables that have a natural zero point (where zero means the absence of the property) and those variables that have zero as an arbitrary point. For example, weight and length have a natural zero point, whereas temperature in degrees Celsius or Fahrenheit has an arbitrary zero point. Variables with a natural zero point are also called *ratio variables*. In statistical practice, however, ratio variables are subjected to operations that treat them as interval and ignore their ratio properties. Therefore, in practice there is no distinction between these two types.

Discrete or continuous?

Here we enter a maze of terminology and its uses and abuses. Let us start with the least controversial aspect. Nominal and ordinal measures are also commonly referred to as categorical variables. They are always discrete. Provided that the categories of a nominal or ordinal variable are exhaustive (cover all potential categories) and mutually exclusive (cases can belong to only one category) then they are naturally discrete in that a case is assigned to a category with no other options. Interval level measures can either be discrete or continuous. For example, number of children is interval level but discrete in that the answers can only be 0, 1, 2, 3, . . . and not 0.6 or 1.34. Age is an interval level measure that is continuous in that someone can actually be one minute or even one second older than someone else. But here is the twist – even if it is a truly continuous phenomenon, we usually measure it in a discrete way! Age is usually in whole years at the last birthday: 12, 13, 14, etc. If you want to think a bit more deeply about it, think about time. Even if we recorded the duration of some event to the nearest tenth of a second – usually not the case in social and behavioural sciences – then it is still a discrete measure because an event could be 23.1657 seconds.

So, let's accept that more often than not we measure continuous phenomena in a discrete way, and these discrete categories such as age last birthday have a standard unit of 1 year between them. How many interval level variables that we commonly use have truly standard units? Age, number of children, time and income are relatively straightforward, but how about all these scales we create from questionnaire items or standard 'instruments' such as the General Health Questionnaire and many other measures of psychological well-being and quality of life? Are the scores from these scales truly interval in that the difference in psychological well-being, for example, is the same between those scoring 4 and those scoring 5 as between those scoring 13 and those scoring 14? Or is there any real difference between those scoring 4 or 5 anyway? It is very common (we do it regularly) to make the assumption that these scales have standard units so that they can be analysed as interval level measures. In general, there is nothing wrong with making this assumption and we would be very restricted in the analysis we could do if we didn't, but it is worth revisiting the basic assumptions we often make in data analysis.

We conclude by summarizing the properties of the various levels of measurement in a table.

▶

Properties of levels of measurement

	Exhaustive	Mutually exclusive	Ordered (rank)	Standard units	Meaningful zero
Nominal	yes	yes	no	no	no
Ordinal	yes	yes	yes	no	no
Interval	yes	yes	yes	yes	no
Ratio	yes	yes	yes	yes	yes

Adapted from Frankfort-Nachmias and Leon-Guerrero (2000: 13–14) and Bowling (2002: 144–7).

At the end of this chapter we examine some of the graphing abilities of Stata and cover some basic single-variable graphs.

FREQUENCY DISTRIBUTIONS

For frequency distributions, you use the **tabulate** command (which you can shorten to **tab** or **ta**). This command will show you the value labels associated with the variable, the frequency of each value, percentage frequency, and cumulative percentage frequency. For example:

tab sex

```
. tab sex

        sex |      Freq.     Percent        Cum.
------------+-----------------------------------
       male |      4,833       47.09       47.09
     female |      5,431       52.91      100.00
------------+-----------------------------------
      Total |     10,264      100.00
```

You will notice that this command gives the value labels, but not the numerical value associated with the label. In order to get that, you must add the option **nolabel** (**nol**) to the **tab** command:

tab sex, nol

```
. tab sex,nol
          sex |      Freq.     Percent        Cum.
--------------+-----------------------------------
            1 |      4,833       47.09       47.09
            2 |      5,431       52.91      100.00
--------------+-----------------------------------
        Total |     10,264      100.00
```

The option **missing** (or **miss** or **m**) gives you information on the missing values.

ta hlstat, miss

```
. ta hlstat,miss
  health over |
last 12 months |      Freq.     Percent        Cum.
--------------+-----------------------------------
    excellent |      2,930       28.55       28.55
         good |      4,613       44.94       73.49
         fair |      1,853       18.05       91.54
         poor |        641        6.25       97.79
    very poor |        219        2.13       99.92
            . |          8        0.08      100.00
--------------+-----------------------------------
        Total |     10,264      100.00
```

The frequency table produced by Stata has three columns of figures. The left-hand one labelled Freq. has the actual counts in each of the categories of the variable. The middle column labelled Percent gives the percentage of that category so that all categories add up to 100%. Note here that when you use the **missing** option the missing-values category contributes to the 100% total so that the percentage is of all cases in your data. If the **missing** option is not used then the percentage is of the number of cases who answered that item – sometimes less than 100% of the total sample. The *hlstat* variable has only eight missing cases, but it could be much higher so that the percentages of the non-missing categories would be inaccurate. See the example below with the *jbsat1* variable. The right-hand column labelled

Cum. gives the cumulative percentage of the categories from the top of the table. The same inclusion rule applies when using the **missing** option.

```
. tab jbsat1,miss

          job |
 satisfaction: |
    promotion |
    prospects |      Freq.     Percent        Cum.
---------------+---------------------------------
 does't apply |        599        5.84        5.84
 not satisfied |       770        7.50       13.34
            2 |        208        2.03       15.36
            3 |        288        2.81       18.17
 not satis/dissat |  1,335       13.01       31.18
            5 |        527        5.13       36.31
            6 |        428        4.17       40.48
 completely satis |    985        9.60       50.08
            . |      5,124       49.92      100.00
---------------+---------------------------------
        Total |     10,264      100.00
```

```
. tab jbsat1

          job |
 satisfaction: |
    promotion |
    prospects |      Freq.     Percent        Cum.
---------------+---------------------------------
 doesn't apply |       599       11.65       11.65
 not satisfied |       770       14.98       26.63
            2 |        208        4.05       30.68
            3 |        288        5.60       36.28
 not satis/dissat |  1,335       25.97       62.26
            5 |        527       10.25       72.51
            6 |        428        8.33       80.84
 completely satis |    985       19.16      100.00
---------------+---------------------------------
        Total |      5,140      100.00
```

In the first table above the **missing** option is used. From this table you might (incorrectly) read that 9.6% are completely satisfied with their promotion prospects. However, when the missing cases are omitted from the second table above, 19.16% are completely satisfied with their promotion prospects. Almost half the total sample was not asked this item because they were not in employment at the time.

Two other options to use with the **tab** command are **plot** and **sort**. The **plot** option produces a basic bar chart of the relative frequencies of the variable categories. This chart is shown in the Results window and not through the graphing facility in Stata. The **sort** option rearranges the frequency table so that the categories are presented in descending order with the most frequent (mode) at the top of the table. These two options can be used together:

tab hlstat, sort plot

```
. tab hlstat, sort plot
    health over |
last 12 months |    Freq.
---------------+---------+--------------------
           good |    4,613 |********************
      excellent |    2,930 |****************
           fair |    1,853 |************
           poor |      641 |*******
      very poor |      219 |**
---------------+---------+--------------------
          Total |   10,256
```

Compare this output with the frequency table given above for the variable *hlstat*. Using the **plot** option will mean that the percentages, category and cumulative, are not presented in the table but using the **sort** option by itself produces the same style of table as earlier by reordered categories.

tab hlstat, sort

```
. tab hlstat, sort

     health over |
 last 12 months |      Freq.     Percent        Cum.
-----------------+-----------------------------------
           good |      4,613       44.98       44.98
      excellent |      2,930       28.57       73.55
           fair |      1,853       18.07       91.61
           poor |        641        6.25       97.86
      very poor |        219        2.14      100.00
-----------------+-----------------------------------
          Total |     10,256      100.00
```

The last two options we will cover here are **nofreq** and **gen**. The **nofreq** option tells Stata not to present the frequencies, which in a single-variable table means that no table is produced. This option has more uses in two-way tables (or crosstabulations) and is covered in the next chapter. The **tab** command combined with the **gen** option produces a series of dummy (or binary) variables – one for every category of the variable in the table. After **gen** goes the name prefix (or stub) of the new series of dummy variables:

tab hlstat,gen(hlth)

The table output is the same as using just the **tab** command but Stata has generated five new variables all starting with *hlth* and called *hlth1*, *hlth2*, *hlth3*, *hlth4* and *hlth5*. These new variables are shown at the bottom of the list of variables in the Variables window. If you **tab** the new variable *hlth3* you can see that the same number of cases (1853) are given the value 1 as were in the third category (fair) on the *hlstat* variable:

tab hlth3

```
. tab hlth3

    hlstat==fai |
              r |      Freq.     Percent        Cum.
-----------------+-----------------------------------
              0 |      8,403       81.93       81.93
              1 |      1,853       18.07      100.00
-----------------+-----------------------------------
          Total |     10,256      100.00
```

Note that if cases are missing on the original variable (*hlstat*) then they will have missing values on these new dummy variables as well.

If you want to use the **tab** command to create a series of dummy variables but do not want to produce a frequency table, then you could use the **gen** and **nofreq** options together:

```
tab hlstat,gen(hlth) nofreq
```

This combination creates the new dummy variables but does not produce a frequency table in the Results window.

If you ask Stata to produce a frequency table of a variable that has a large number of categories/values then it will return an error message in red: too many values

The **if** qualifier works with almost all commands, including recoding and variable creation. Try:

```
tab hlstat if sex==1
```

This command gives you the frequency distribution of health status for males. Don't forget that double equals signs are required for conditional commands like this.

Alternatively, the **bysort** command can be combined with **tab**. For example, the command below will produce two frequency tables – one for the health status for males and one for health status of females. The **missing, nolabel, plot** and **sort** options can still be used in this combination.

```
bysort sex: tab mastat
```

```
. bysort sex:tab hlstat

-----------------------------------------------------------
-> sex = male

      health over |
   last 12 months |     Freq.    Percent        Cum.
------------------+-----------------------------------
        excellent |     1,536      31.79       31.79
             good |     2,149      44.47       76.26
             fair |       808      16.72       92.98
             poor |       246       5.09       98.08
        very poor |        93       1.92      100.00
------------------+-----------------------------------
            Total |     4,832     100.00
```

```
-------------------------------------------------
-> sex = female

   health over |
last 12 months |    Freq.   Percent        Cum.
---------------+---------------------------------
     excellent |    1,394     25.70        25.70
          good |    2,464     45.43        71.13
          fair |    1,045     19.27        90.39
          poor |      395      7.28        97.68
     very poor |      126      2.32       100.00
---------------+---------------------------------
         Total |    5,424    100.00
```

If you want to produce a series of frequency tables you do not need to type in each **tab** command separately. The command **tab1** will produce separate frequency tables for each of the variables in the list after the command. For example: **tab1 sex hlstat** will produce a frequency table for *sex* followed by one for *hlstat*. The variable list can, of course, be much longer.

```
. tab1 sex hlstat

-> tabulation of sex

           sex |    Freq.   Percent        Cum.
---------------+---------------------------------
          male |    4,833     47.09        47.09
        female |    5,431     52.91       100.00
---------------+---------------------------------
         Total |   10,264    100.00


-> tabulation of hlstat

   health over |
last 12 months |    Freq.   Percent        Cum.
---------------+---------------------------------
     excellent |    2,930     28.57        28.57
          good |    4,613     44.98        73.55
          fair |    1,853     18.07        91.61
          poor |      641      6.25        97.86
     very poor |      219      2.14       100.00
---------------+---------------------------------
         Total |   10,256    100.00
```

The options **nolabel, missing, sort** and **nofreq** can be used with the **tab1** command as well. The **gen** option can also be used but care needs to be taken as the category values from the original variables will be used, but if the values are duplicated then Stata will stop and send an error message as it will not create two variables with the same name. Our advice is to use the **gen** option only with single-variable tabulations.

Frequency tables can also be produced by using the pull-down menus (see Box 5.2).

Box 5.2: Frequency tables using pull-down menus

Although we advocate quick progress to using do files and we use single interactive commands in the Command window in this and other chapters, Stata has the facility to use pull-down menus. You can also use these to produce descriptive statistics in frequency tables and summary statistics.

Statistics → Summaries, tables, and tests → Tables → One-way tables

This path shows that you need to first choose the **Statistics** main pull down menu from the top toolbar then follow the blue sub menus to **One-way tables**.

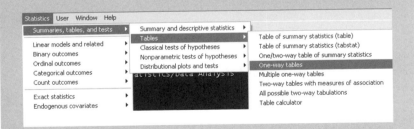

This brings up the dialogue box called **tabulate 1 - one-way tables**. This dialogue box has four tabs: **Main, by/if/in, Weights** and **Advanced**.

On the **Main** tab, use the list of variables under the **Categorical variable** selector to choose the variable you want to put into a frequency table – in this case the variable *sex*.

▶

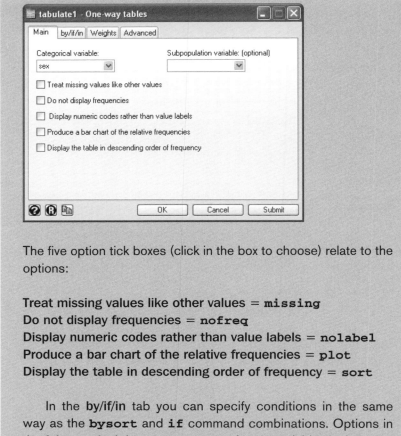

The five option tick boxes (click in the box to choose) relate to the options:

Treat missing values like other values = `missing`
Do not display frequencies = `nofreq`
Display numeric codes rather than value labels = `nolabel`
Produce a bar chart of the relative frequencies = `plot`
Display the table in descending order of frequency = `sort`

In the **by/if/in** tab you can specify conditions in the same way as the **bysort** and **if** command combinations. Options in the **Advanced** tab let you create new dummy variables in the same way as the **gen** option.

SUMMARY STATISTICS

The command for common summary statistics is **summarize**, which can be shortened to **sum** or **su**. The command is followed by the variable or list of variables you wish to analyse.

Be careful, because just typing **sum** in the Command window will produce summary statistics of all the variables in the data, which can result in pages and pages of output if you have a very large data set! If you find you have done this – or made any other mistake where Stata ends up returning far too much information – you can always click on the **Break** button ⊗ to stop the command.

The **sum** command produces basic descriptive statistics such as the number of observations (Obs), mean, standard deviation (Std. Dev.), minimum and maximum values. For example:

sum ghqscale

```
. sum ghqscale

Variable |     Obs        Mean    Std. Dev.   Min   Max
---------+-------------------------------------------
ghqscale |    9613    10.77125    4.914182     0    36
```

Additional statistics can be obtained by adding the **detail** option:

sum ghqscale, detail

```
. sum ghqscale, detail

              subjective wellbeing (ghq) 1: likert
-------------------------------------------------------
      Percentiles   Smallest
 1%          3          0
 5%          5          0
10%          6          0                Obs          9613
25%          7          0    Sum of Wgt.              9613

50%         10                           Mean      10.77125
                         Largest    Std. Dev.      4.914182
75%         13         36
90%         17         36    Variance     24.14919
95%         21         36    Skewness     1.366197
99%         27         36    Kurtosis     5.713574
```

This expanded output includes information on the number of cases, mean and standard deviation. The minimum and maximum values can be seen with the percentile listing on the left. The 50th percentile (median) is also reported here along with the 25th and 75th percentiles for the inter-quartile range. The variance (standard deviation squared) is presented in the right-hand column along with statistics for the skewness and kurtosis of the variable (see Box 5.3).

Box 5.3: Skewness and kurtosis

The skewness statistic summarizes the degree and direction of asymmetry in the distribution of the variable. A symmetric distribution has a skewness statistic of 0. If the distribution is skewed to the left (or negatively skewed) the statistic has a negative value, and if the distribution is skewed to the right (or positively skewed) the statistic has a positive value. In the above example, the skewness has a value of 1.37 indicating that the distribution of the GHQ variable is skewed to the right. We will revisit this distribution later in the chapter when we look at graphing.

The kurtosis statistic is a summary of the shape of the distribution in relation to its peak and tails. A normal distribution has a kurtosis of 3. If the value is less than 3 then the distribution is 'flatter' than a normal distribution, with a lower peak and heavier or wider tails. If the value is greater than 3 then the distribution is 'sharper' than a normal distribution, with a higher peak and lighter or narrower tails. In this example of the *ghqscale* variable the kurtosis statistic has a value of 5.71 indicating that it is more peaked than normal, with thinner tails.

Other software calculates skewness and kurtosis statistics differently, so you need to make sure you know how the statistics are calculated so you can interpret them correctly.

In Stata you can also use the **sktest** command to formally test the normality of a variable. Two other commands – **swilk** and **sfrancia** – are also available depending on the sample size. The **sktest** command tests the skewness and kurtosis of the variable with a null hypothesis that the variable is normally distributed. Our examination of the *ghqscale* variable shows that we would reject the null hypothesis on both its skewness and kurtosis. Note that the **sktest** command does not produce the value of the statistics, and you would need to run a summary statistics command to obtain the actual values.

```
. sktest ghqscale

          Skewness/Kurtosis tests for Normality

                                        ----- joint -----
Variable |  Pr(Skewness)  Pr(Kurtosis)  adj chi2(2)  Prob>chi2
---------+---------------------------------------------------
ghqscale |      0.000         0.000           .           .
```

The **sum** command and **detail** option can be used with more than one variable. Without the **detail** option, Stata produces a list of the variables with separating lines after every fifth variable. For example:

sum ghqa-ghql

```
. sum ghqa-ghql
```

Variable	Obs	Mean	Std. Dev.	Min	Max
ghqa	9728	2.162212	.5286127	1	4
ghqb	9728	1.7978	.778507	1	4
ghqc	9719	2.049079	.5911111	1	4
ghqd	9730	1.969476	.4843033	1	4
ghqe	9729	2.058999	.7992425	1	4
ghqf	9718	1.760136	.7077888	1	4
ghqg	9730	2.131449	.5690908	1	4
ghqh	9732	2.02949	.4746731	1	4
ghqi	9730	1.854265	.8214758	1	4
ghqj	9687	1.597399	.7404045	1	4
ghqk	9677	1.361992	.6329897	1	4
ghql	9684	2.011669	.5338565	1	4

The separating lines can be omitted by using the **sep(0)** option and changed to any other interval you wish; for example, for an interval of variables use **sep(2)**:

sum ghqa-ghql, sep(2)

```
. sum ghqa- ghql,sep(2)
```

Variable	Obs	Mean	Std. Dev.	Min	Max
ghqa	9728	2.162212	.5286127	1	4
ghqb	9728	1.7978	.778507	1	4
ghqc	9719	2.049079	.5911111	1	4
ghqd	9730	1.969476	.4843033	1	4
ghqe	9729	2.058999	.7992425	1	4
ghqf	9718	1.760136	.7077888	1	4

```
--------+--------------------------------------
   ghqg |   9730   2.131449    .5690908    1    4
   ghqh |   9732   2.02949     .4746731    1    4
--------+--------------------------------------
   ghqi |   9730   1.854265    .8214758    1    4
   ghqj |   9687   1.597399    .7404045    1    4
--------+--------------------------------------
   ghqk |   9677   1.361992    .6329897    1    4
   ghql |   9684   2.011669    .5338565    1    4
```

As we have mentioned before, there are usually a few different ways of producing the statistics you want in Stata so there is some overlap with the following commands. The style of presentation differs, and for some commands this can be adjusted to suit your preferences.

If you wish to produce the standard error of the mean and confidence intervals instead of the standard deviation, minimum and maximum values you can use the **ci** command.

ci ghqscale

```
. ci ghqscale

Variable |   Obs      Mean   Std. Err.   [95% Conf. Interval]
---------+---------------------------------------------------
ghqscale |   9613   10.77125   .0501212    10.673  10.8695
```

The default output shows the number of cases (Obs) and mean as with the **sum** command, but then the standard error of the mean (Std. Err.) and 95% confidence interval are shown. The level of the confidence intervals can be chosen by using the **level** option. For example, if you wanted the 99% confidence intervals:

ci ghqscale, level(99)

```
. ci ghqscale,level(99)

Variable |   Obs      Mean   Std. Err.   [99% Conf. Interval]
---------+---------------------------------------------------
ghqscale |   9613   10.77125   .0501212    10.64212  10.90038
```

The **mean** command produces similar output to the default **ci** command and also has the **level** option. The other options for

mean enable you to specify how the standard error is calculated using jackknife, bootstrap or clustering adjustments.

```
. mean ghqscale

Mean estimation                      Number of obs = 9613
--------------------------------------------------------
         |       Mean   Std. Err.  [95% Conf. Interval]
---------+----------------------------------------------
ghqscale | 10.77125   .0501212        10.673 10.8695
--------------------------------------------------------
```

The command **ameans** will produce the arithmetic, geometric and harmonic means with confidence intervals for the variables listed.

```
. ameans ghqscale

Variable |       Type   Obs     Mean  [95% Conf. Interval]
---------+------------------------------------------------
ghqscale | Arithmetic  9613  10.77125     10.673   10.8695
         |  Geometric  9602  9.802626   9.716335 9.889682
         |   Harmonic  9602  8.825263   8.724163 8.928735
         --------------------------------------------------
```

An extremely useful and flexible command for producing descriptive or summary statistics is **tabstat**. This command can also be used extensively when summarizing variables by categories of another variable, and this use is covered in Chapter 6.

If you use just the **tabstat** command without any options then Stata simply returns the mean. However, the **tabstat** command can produce a large number of statistics. In the output below **tabstat** is used first on its own and then with a **statistics** option (shortened to **s**) that specifies the number of cases (**n**), mean (**me**), standard deviation (**sd**), minimum value (**min**) and maximum value (**max**). This second output is similar to that produced by the **sum** command.

```
. tabstat ghqscale

variable |        mean
---------+----------
ghqscale |   10.77125
---------------------
```

```
. tabstat ghqscale,s(n me sd min max)

variable |        N       mean         sd   min   max
---------+------------------------------------------
ghqscale |     9613  10.77125   4.914182     0    36
---------+------------------------------------------
```

The **statistics** or **s** option can be used to generate other summary statistics and the output will be in the order specified inside the parentheses of the option. In this example Stata has produced the number of cases, mean and standard deviation, followed by the standard error of the mean (**sem**), skewness (**sk**) and kurtosis (**kur**). You may wish to compare this style of output with that produced by **sum** and the **detail** option.

```
. tabstat ghqscale,s(n me sd sem sk kur)

variable |     N     mean       sd se(mean) skewness kurtosis
---------+---------------------------------------------------
ghqscale |  9613 10.77125 4.914182 .0501212 1.366197 5.713574
---------+---------------------------------------------------
```

The default style of output of the **tabstat** command with only one variable is to put the requested statistics in one row as in the above example. However, if you are specifying a large number of statistics you may find it more convenient to have them in a column. This can be done by using a **column(variable)** option which can be shortened to **c(v)**. In the example below additional statistics have been requested. These are inter-quartile range (**iqr**) and quartiles (**q**) which includes the median (p50 in the output). The median could be requested on its own by using **med** in the statistics option brackets.

```
. tabstat ghqscale,s(n me sd sem sk kur iqr q) c(v)

    stats |  ghqscale
---------+----------
        N |      9613
     mean |  10.77125
       sd |  4.914182
 se(mean) |  .0501212
 skewness |  1.366197
 kurtosis |  5.713574
      iqr |         6
      p25 |         7
      p50 |        10
      p75 |        13
---------+----------
```

One odd feature of the **tabstat** command is that when you have two or more variables the default output is to put the variables in columns. Three variables are shown in this example. So, for two or more variables, if you want the statistics to be presented in rows then you need to use the **column(statistic)** option – shortened to **c(s)** – to produce the second output below.

```
. tabstat ghqa-ghqc,s(n me sd min max)

    stats |        ghqa        ghqb        ghqc
 ---------+---------------------------------------
        N |        9728        9728        9719
     mean |    2.162212      1.7978    2.049079
       sd |     .5286127     .778507    .5911111
      min |           1           1           1
      max |           4           4           4
 ---------------------------------------------------
```

```
. tabstat ghqa-ghqc,s(n me sd min max) c(s)

 variable |      N       mean         sd   min   max
 ---------+---------------------------------------------
     ghqa |   9728   2.162212    .5286127     1     4
     ghqb |   9728     1.7978     .778507     1     4
     ghqc |   9719   2.049079    .5911111     1     4
 ------------------------------------------------------
```

All of the summary statistics commands – **sum, mean, ci, ameans** and **tabstat** – can be combined with **bysort** and **if** commands. For example, if you wanted the summary statistics for these three variables, but separately for men and women, then you could use the **bysort** command.

```
. bysort sex: tabstat ghqa-ghqc,s(n me sk)

 ----------------------------------------------------
 -> sex = male

    stats |        ghqa        ghqb        ghqc
 ---------+---------------------------------------
        N |        4522        4523        4521
     mean |    2.125387    1.688702    2.040478
 skewness |    1.094095    .9064145    .8466639
 ---------------------------------------------------
```

```
------------------------------------------------
-> sex = female

    stats |         ghqa         ghqb         ghqc
----------+-------------------------------------
        N |         5206         5205         5198
     mean |     2.194199     1.892603      2.05656
 skewness |     1.134487      .6264102     1.016004
------------------------------------------------
```

However, the **tabstat** command has a **by** option that you can use to specify output split by categories of another variable. The advantage of using the **by** option is that the summary statistics for the total sample are also produced. The output below comes from the **by** option and you can see that the male and female summary statistics are given above the total sample statistics.

```
. tabstat ghqa-ghqc,s(n me sk) by(sex)
```

Summary statistics: N, mean, skewness
    by categories of: sex (sex)

```
      sex |         ghqa         ghqb         ghqc
----------+-------------------------------------
     male |         4522         4523         4521
          |     2.125387     1.688702     2.040478
          |     1.094095      .9064145      .8466639
----------+-------------------------------------
   female |         5206         5205         5198
          |     2.194199     1.892603      2.05656
          |     1.134487      .6264102     1.016004
----------+-------------------------------------
    Total |         9728         9728         9719
          |     2.162212       1.7978     2.049079
          |      1.10933      .7433614      .932651
------------------------------------------------
```

Summary statistics can also be produced using the pull-down menus (see Box 5.4).

Box 5.4: Summary statistics using pull-down menus

The path:

Statistics → Summaries, tables, and tests → Summary and descriptive statistics → Summary statistics

takes you to a dialogue box called **summarize - Summary statistics**. It has three tabs. In the **Main** tab you enter the variables you want statistics for by either typing them into the **Variables** box or by scrolling through the list of all variables and selecting the ones you want.

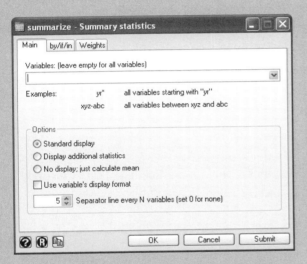

If you select the **Display additional statistics** option then Stata will present the same output as the `detail` option. In the **by/if/in** tab you can specify conditions in the same way as the `bysort` and `if` command combinations.

This path will take you to a dialogue box equivalent to the **means** command:

Statistics → Summaries, tables, and tests → Summary and descriptive statistics → Means

The variables are entered as before in the **Model** tab, with command combinations in the **if/in/over** tab. The **SE/Cluster** tab allows you to specify the type of standard error calculation appropriate

▶

▶ for your data. The **Reporting** tab allows you to specify confidence intervals other than the default 95%.

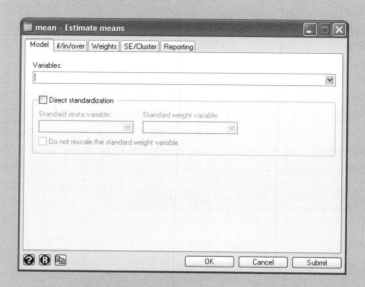

This path takes you to a dialogue box equivalent to the `ci` command:

Statistics → Summaries, tables, and tests → Summary and descriptive statistics → Confidence intervals

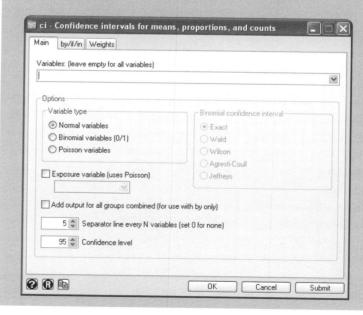

GRAPHS

The graphing facilities in Stata have improved significantly since version 6 and now Stata is able to produce publication-quality graphics. The downside is that the commands have become more complicated and sometimes extend to two or three lines (often more), and the graphics now have their own manual. Rather than try and cover all the command options and structure, experience has taught us that it is better to use the pull-down menus to introduce graphing in Stata, much as it goes against our aim to get you using do files as soon as possible. In version 9 there is a **Graphics** pull-down menu function called **Easy graphs** which was removed in version 10, but the functions are retained in other menus. Here we cover using the main graph functions in the **Graphics** pull-down menu in version 10. If you are using version 9, then see Box 5.5 for an introduction to the use of **Easy graphs**.

Box 5.5: Easy graphs **in version 9**

The path through the pull-down menus is:

Graphics → Easy graphs

This opens a full list of graphing options:

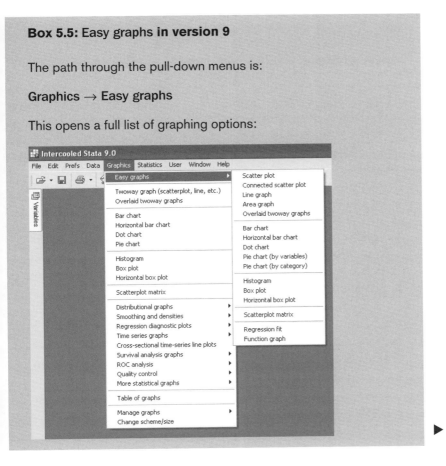

▶   **Pie charts**

Graphics → Easy graphs → Pie chart (by category)

This path will take you to a dialogue box called **graph pie - Pie chart (by category)** where you enter the variable name for which you want to graph the categories. The pie chart produced from the default settings can be a little messy and may need tidying up before it is ready for a report.

Box plots

Graphics → Easy graphs → Box plot
Graphics → Easy graphs → Horizontal box plot

The box plot can either be vertical or horizontal depending on its use and your preference.

Histograms

Graphics → Easy graphs → Histogram

The pull-down menu takes you to a dialogue box called **histogram - Histogram for continuous and categorical variables**. In the **Main** tab you can either type in or scroll down the list of variables in the **Variable** box. On the right-hand side you select whether the variable chosen is either continuous or discrete. If you want the histogram to display percentages instead of the default density scale on the Y axis you select the **Options** tab and select **Percent** in the **Y axis** box on the lower left-hand side. The level of information given is probably enough to judge the distribution but falls well short of report quality. Note that the default is that the bars still touch even for discrete variables, which many would consider to be technically incorrect.

For continuous variables, after typing in or selecting the variable, select the **Continuous data** option in the **Main** tab. In the **Options** tab you can tick the **Add normal density plot** option in the **Density plot options** box on the right-hand side. This will show a normal distribution for the same mean and standard deviation as the variable so you can compare the actual distribution with an expected normal distribution.

The default graph format and colours are determined by the graph preferences through the pull-down menu path

Edit → **Preferences** → **Graph Preferences**

This brings up a box that shows that the default scheme is s2 color and the default font is Arial. If you prefer your graphs to be formatted differently then you can change these. Stata has numerous schemes to choose from. Once set in this box, every future graph will be formatted in this way. However, each individual graph scheme and fonts can be changed in the tabs when you are creating the graph and you should check that what you are choosing is consistent with the general scheme.

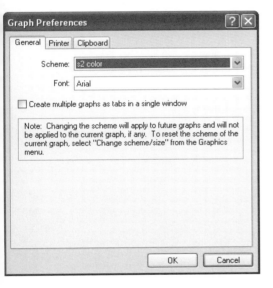

When you create a graph it opens in a new window. You can leave this window open while you return to Stata (by clicking anywhere in the main Stata windows), but then the graph is not shown. On the toolbar there is an icon – 🖼 · in version 9 and ᴸᵃ · in version 10 – that will bring the graph back to the front. The icon is dimmed when there isn't a graph to show.

The biggest, and best, change in version 10 is the interactive graphics editor. To open the editor you need to right-click on the **Graph** window and select **Start Graph Editor** or click on this icon 🖼 on the toolbar above the graph when it's first created (see Box 5.6). You can do this at any time a graph window is open.

The editor is very powerful and very intuitive and it allows you, for example, to easily add text and arrows to more clearly indicate what the graph is showing, as well as format the graph, axes, and titles. The Stata website says that you should get the hang of it in a few minutes as you just click on what you want to change; they are right. It's easy to get the hang of and makes many of the options available in the tabs unnecessary to start with as you can change them in the Graph Editor. Try creating basic graphs and then editing them. For a detailed text on Stata graphics, see Mitchell (2008).

Box 5.6: Graphs and the Graph Editor

When you first create a graph it opens in a window called **Stata Graph - Graph** as shown below for a histogram of the GHQ. If this graph is what you want to save or copy then you can do this from the pull-down menus or using the icons on the toolbar. If you wish to use the Graph Editor then click on the ▨ icon on the toolbar.

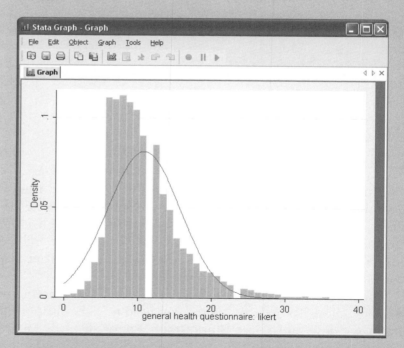

This opens the Graph Editor which looks like this. Note here that you cannot do any data analysis in Stata while the Graph Editor is open. If you need to do this then save the graph (see Box 5.7) and return to editing the graph after your analysis. To edit an area of the graph either click on it with the cursor or click on the part in the list on the right-hand side.

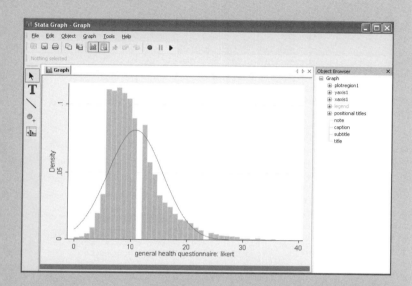

For example, if we wanted to change the X axis title we could (a) double-click on the title **general health questionnaire: likert** or (b) click on the + symbol next to xaxis1 in the **Object Browser** on the right of the Editor. This expands to show the title in the tree, then double-click on **title**.

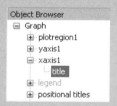

Both of these will bring up a new window where you can change the text, font, colour and position. If you are not exactly sure what the changes will look like we suggest you click on the **Apply** button which will keep this window open while you can see the changes in the graph. Once you are happy with the changes then click on the **OK** button to close this window.

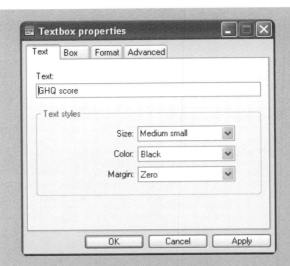

After changing the X axis title and adding a main title, caption and some text the final graph looks much more informative. You can see that as the text box and arrow have been added, the tree in the **Object Browser** has expanded to include **added text** and **added lines** which you can double-click on to edit. Above the graph on the left you can see a tab with **Graph*** on it. This is the name of the graph – at this stage we haven't saved it – and the * tells you that it has been changed since it was last saved.

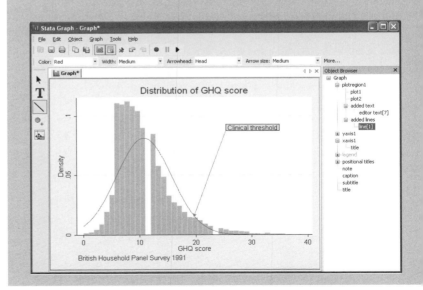

The **Graphics** pull-down menu has numerous choices, but in this chapter we will introduce some of the basic single-variable graphs: pie charts, box plots and histograms. The histograms in Stata cover both continuous and discrete variables. We cover two-way, or two-variable, graphs in Chapter 6.

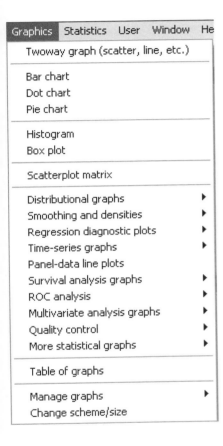

PIE CHARTS

Graphics → Pie chart

This path will take you to a dialogue box called **graph pie - Pie charts** where, in the **Main** tab, you enter the variable name for which you want to graph the categories. Pie charts are most appropriate for variables that have relatively few categories as they are better displayed and interpreted. In this example we use the *hlstat* variable. We click on **Graph by categories** as we want to see the categories of the variable.

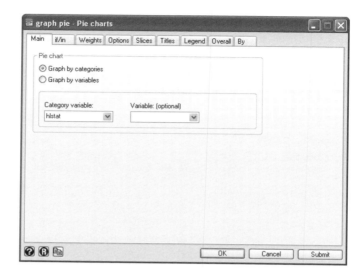

You can either type in the variable name or use the down arrow to scroll through the list of variables and select one. The **if/in** tab allows you to specify that the graph is to be based on a subset of cases. The **Titles** tab gives a number of options for titles and labels on the graph. The **Options** tab is where you can change the colour scheme.

The pie chart produced below is from these settings and some minor editing in the **Graph Editor**; it is still a little messy and would need tidying up before it is ready for a report.

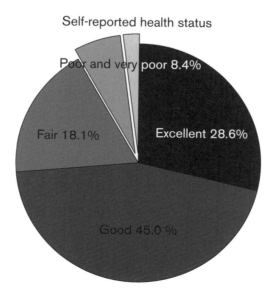

BOX PLOTS

Graphics → **Box plot**

Box plots (or box-and-whisker plots) are a good way to examine the distribution of a variable(s). The distribution is shown against an axis of the values of the variable. The box plot can either be vertical or horizontal depending on its use and your preferences.

The pull-down menu path takes you to a dialogue box titled **graph box - Box plots** which has a **Variables** box where you can either type or scroll through and select variable(s). For now we concentrate on single-variable plots. There are other tabs in this window. The **Categories** tab is where you specify categorical variables to produce box plots to compare, and this is covered in more detail in the next chapter. The **if/in** tab allows you to specify that the graph is to be based on a subset of cases. The **Titles** tab gives a number of options for titles and labels on the graph. The **Options** tab is where you can change the colour scheme and choose how to treat missing values.

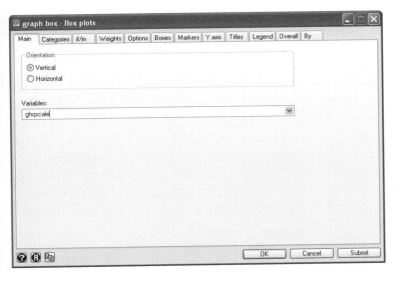

Box plots are normally used for interval level (or continuous) variables and are not appropriate for ordinal or nominal level variables. In this example we want to graph the variable *ghqscale* so we enter this in the **Variables** box and select **OK**.

The box in the box plot shows the inter-quartile range; that is, the values from the 25th to the 75th percentile. The line in the middle of the box is the median or 50th percentile. The whiskers show the lower and upper adjacent values. These are the furthest observations which are within 1.5 times the inter-quartile range of the lower and upper ends of the box. If you wish to check these figures you can see the earlier results from the **su ghqscale, detail** command.

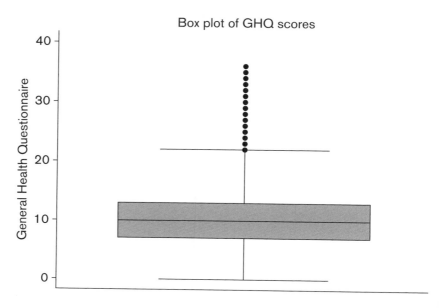

In this example the median is 10, with the 25th percentile being 7 and the 75th percentile being 13. This makes the inter-quartile range $13 - 7 = 6$. Therefore, the upper whisker is $1.5 \times 6 = 9$ from the 75th percentile, which is $13 + 9 = 22$. All cases that have GHQ scores higher than 22 are potential outliers and are shown in the box plot as dots. The lower whisker extends to zero (the minimum value of the variable) because the 25th percentile is 7; subtracting 1.5 times the interquartile range gives -2, which is not a possible value.

From this box plot you might conclude that the *ghqscale* variable is slightly skewed to the right (or positively skewed) as there a number of outliers above the upper whisker.

If you wish to produce a series of box plots for two or more variables then you can enter two or more variables in the **Variables** box on the **Main** tab. In the example below we have added the *age* variable to the *ghqscale* variable. Stata produces the two plots side by side. Note that Stata uses the variable labels as they are in the data set so good labels are useful, but with a quick use of the Graph Editor you can easily change them into more meaningful labels if necessary. You need to be careful when choosing variables to graph together because if one has a very small range compared to the other then the plot will be so compressed that judging its distribution will be difficult.

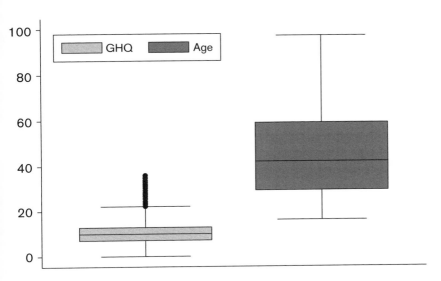

HISTOGRAMS

Graphics → Histogram

Histograms are the most common way of visually inspecting the distribution of a variable. However, there is a minefield of discipline-specific terminology to negotiate when using histograms and/or bar charts (bar graphs). For bar charts in Stata, see Chapter 6.

The main characteristic of a 'pure' histogram is that the area of the bars represents the value of the data, which is why the default scale for the Y axis in Stata graphs is density. The density means that the heights of the bars are adjusted so that the sum of their areas equals 1, as the width of the bars are the same for each category. As many users prefer to see the Y axis scaled in other ways, Stata offers three further options:

- Fraction: the height of all the bars equals 1.
- Frequency: the height of the bars is equal to the number of observations in the category.
- Percent: the height of all the bars equals 100.

One of the main distinctions Stata uses in constructing histograms is whether the variable is continuous (interval) or discrete (ordinal or nominal). For continuous variables Stata can automatically determine the grouping of the values to display in the bars of the chart, but for discrete variables one bar for every category is shown. The number of bars used for continuous variables is an option that we come to later.

In the first example, we use a discrete variable *hlstat*. The pull-down menu takes you to a dialogue box called **histogram - Histograms for continuous and categorical variables**. In the **Main** tab you can either type in or scroll down the list of variables in the **Variable** box. To the right of this you select whether the data chosen is continuous or discrete.

In this case we also want the histogram to display percentages instead of the default density scale on the Y axis so we select **Percent** in the **Y axis** box on the lower left-hand side. We have specified that 'height labels' are added to the bars. As we have asked for the bars to represent percentages, percentages will be shown. You can see that the **Bar properties** button on the lower left has an * on it, which shows that we have asked for some of the bar characteristics to be changed from the default settings. These are to do with presentation as we want the bars to be separated rather than touching, the latter being the default setting.

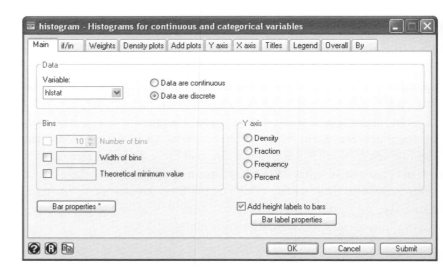

These settings followed by some editing in the Graph Editor produces the histogram shown below.

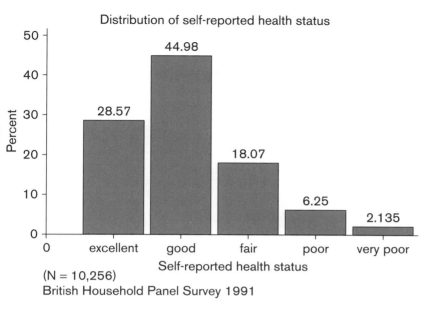

Distribution of self-reported health status

(N = 10,256)
British Household Panel Survey 1991

We follow a similar process in this second example but use a continuous variable *ghqscale* as in the box plot examples above. This time, after typing in or selecting the variable, select the **Continuous data** option in the **Main** tab. We leave the Y axis as the default density scale but we tick the **Add normal density plot** option in the **Density plots** tab. This will show a normal distribution for the same mean and standard deviation as the variable so we can compare the actual distribution with an expected normal distribution.

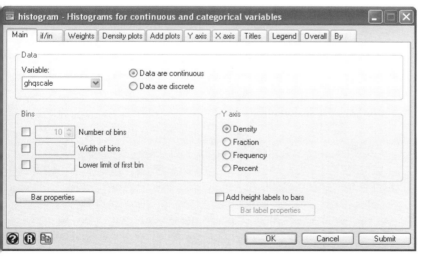

These options will produce the histogram shown below, which will need further editing in order to be of report quality. As you can see from the actual distribution against the expected normal distribution the variable *ghqscale* is slightly skewed to the right, confirming what we saw in the box plots.

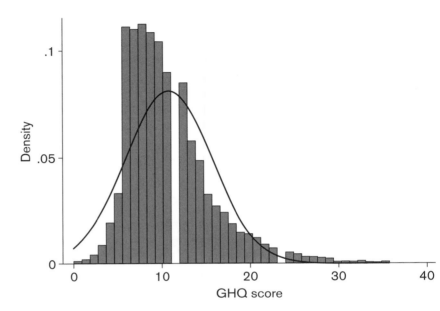

Multiple graphs can also be combined into a single display (see Box 5.7).

Box 5.7: Saving and combining graphs

To save a graph for the first time use the **File** → **Save As** pull-down menu. Then choose where you want to save it by browsing in the usual way. Once the graph has been saved any further changes can be saved by clicking on the disk icon on the toolbar.

Saved graphs can be opened by using the **File** → **Open graph** pull-down menu in the main Stata window or by typing **graph use** "path/graphname" in the Command window.

Rather than displaying single graphs you may want to combine a set of graphs in one image for a report or publication. This is easily done in Stata by using the **graph combine** command. Below is an example of some of the graphs we have created in this chapter combined into one image using the command:

```
graph combine pie.gph box.gph box2.gph ///
    histogram1.gph histogram2.gph
```

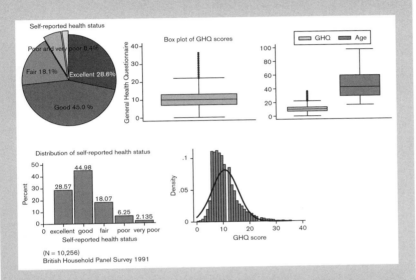

There are options to the **graph combine** command to choose columns or rows and positions. The really nice thing is that the new combined image opens in the Chart Editor so you can edit the image even more to ensure it's exactly what you want.

DEMONSTRATION EXERCISE

In Chapter 3 we manipulated the individual level variables and saved a new data set called demodata1.dta. In Chapter 4 we merged a household level variable indicating the region of the country onto the individual level data and saved the data with a new name demodata2.dta. In this chapter we analyse the variables we are going to use for their distribution, measures of central tendency and, for continuous variables, their normality.

First, we determine the level of measurement of all the variables:

Variable	Level of measurement
female	nominal
age	interval
agecat	ordinal
marst2	nominal
empstat	nominal
numchd	ordinal
region2	nominal
d_ghq	nominal
ghqscale	interval

Starting with the nominal and ordinal level variables, we simply tabulate these to examine the number of cases in each of the categories.

tab1 female agecat marst2 empstat numchd ///
   region2 d_ghq

```
. tab1 female agecat marst2 empstat numchd ///
    region2 d_ghq

-> tabulation of female

      female |
   indicator |      Freq.    Percent       Cum.
-------------+-----------------------------------
        male |      3,914      47.95      47.95
      female |      4,249      52.05     100.00
-------------+-----------------------------------
       Total |      8,163     100.00

-> tabulation of agecat

         age |
  categories |      Freq.    Percent       Cum.
-------------+-----------------------------------
 18-32 years |      2,956      36.21      36.21
 33-50 years |      3,336      40.87      77.08
 51-65 years |      1,871      22.92     100.00
-------------+-----------------------------------
       Total |      8,163     100.00
```

```
-> tabulation of marst2
       marital |
      status 4 |
    categories |    Freq.     Percent        Cum.
---------------+-------------------------------
        single |    1,619       19.83       19.83
       married |    5,786       70.88       90.71
       sep/div |      569        6.97       97.68
       widowed |      189        2.32      100.00
---------------+-------------------------------
         Total |    8,163      100.00

-> tabulation of empstat

    employment |
        status |    Freq.     Percent        Cum.
---------------+-------------------------------
      employed |    5,575       70.89       70.89
    unemployed |      505        6.42       77.31
 longterm sick |      244        3.10       80.42
      studying |      224        2.85       83.27
   family care |      913       11.61       94.88
       retired |      403        5.12      100.00
---------------+-------------------------------
         Total |    7,864      100.00

-> tabulation of numchd

    children 3 |
    categories |    Freq.     Percent        Cum.
---------------+-------------------------------
          none |    5,182       63.48       63.48
    one or two |    2,443       29.93       93.41
  three or more |      538        6.59      100.00
---------------+-------------------------------
         Total |    8,163      100.00
```

```
-> tabulation of region2

         regions 7 |
      categories |  Freq.   Percent      Cum.
------------------+-----------------------------
          London |    898     11.00     11.00
           South |  2,504     30.67     41.68
        Midlands |  1,399     17.14     58.81
       Northwest |    849     10.40     69.21
North and Northeast |  1,310   16.05     85.26
           Wales |    423      5.18     90.44
        Scotland |    780      9.56    100.00
------------------+-----------------------------
           Total |  8,163    100.00
```

```
-> tabulation of d_ghq

          d_ghq |  Freq.   Percent      Cum.
----------------+-----------------------------
             0 |  6,271     81.29     81.29
             1 |  1,443     18.71    100.00
----------------+-----------------------------
         Total |  7,714    100.00
```

For the interval level variables we have a number of options when inspecting them. We start with simple descriptive statistics.

su age ghqscale

```
. su age ghqscale

Variable |    Obs        Mean   Std. Dev.   Min   Max
---------+--------------------------------------------
     age |   8163    39.32733    13.08993    18    65
ghqscale |   7714    10.78727    4.945154     0    36
```

Next, we use the pull-down menus to produce histograms of the two variables with expected normal distributions in order to compare them and judge any skewness. The histograms below show that the distribution of the *age* variable is rather flat compared to the normal distribution, with more cases in the younger ages than the older ones. The distribution of the GHQ variable (*ghqscale*) is more peaked than the expected normal distribution and slightly skewed to the right.

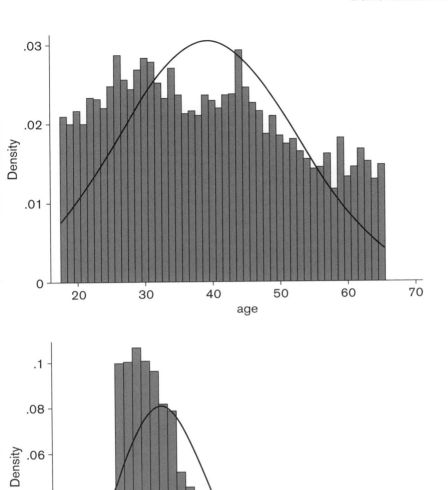

We now use the **tabstat** command to produce summary statistics for these two variables and then test their skewness and kurtosis using the **sktest** command (see Box 5.3).

```
tabstat age ghqscale, s(sk kur)
sktest age ghqscale
```

```
. tabstat age ghqscale, s(sk kur)

    stats |          age    ghqscale
---------+--------------------------
 skewness |    .2223762    1.364399
 kurtosis |    1.981199    5.661401
---------+--------------------------

. sktest age ghqscale

              Skewness/Kurtosis tests for Normality
                                          ----- joint -----
  Variable | Pr(Skewness) Pr(Kurtosis) adj chi2(2) Prob>chi2
---------+---------------------------------------------------
      age |       0.000        0.000           .         .
 ghqscale |       0.000        0.000           .         .
```

From the first part of the output you can see that the *age* variable has a skewness statistic of 0.22 which, being positive, indicates it is slightly skewed to the right, and a kurtosis statistic of 1.98 which, being less than 3, indicates that the distribution is flatter than normal. For the *ghqscale* variable the skewness value of 1.36 indicates that the distribution is skewed to the right and the kurtosis value of 5.66 indicates a distribution more peaked than normal.

Most of the techniques that we will use in this demonstration are robust to reasonable departures from normality such as these, but for the sake of this exercise we will consider what we might do if we wanted to transform the *ghqscale* variable to a distribution closer to normal. For distributions that are skewed to the right, one of the usual transformations used is the logarithmic (either natural logarithm or base 10). However, with this variable there is a problem in that it contains cases that have a score of zero. The logarithmic transformation of zero is not possible as it is minus infinity. You can see this if we transform the variable as it stands.

gen ln_ghq=ln(ghqscale)
su ghqscale ln_ghq

```
. gen ln_ghq=ln(ghqscale)
(459 missing values generated)

. su ghqscale ln_ghq

 Variable |     Obs        Mean    Std. Dev.     Min        Max
---------+---------------------------------------------------------
 ghqscale |    7714    10.78727    4.945154        0         36
   ln_ghq |    7704    2.283492    .4439032        0   3.583519
```

The new variable (*ln_ghq*) has 10 fewer cases than the original variable (*ghqscale*). This is because there were ten cases with a value of zero in the *ghqscale* variable. This can be checked by either:

tab ghqscale if ghqscale<2

or

count if ghqscale==0

```
. ta ghqscale if ghqscale<2

  ghq 0-36 |     Freq.     Percent        Cum.
-----------+-----------------------------------
         0 |        10       40.00       40.00
         1 |        15       60.00      100.00
-----------+-----------------------------------
     Total |        25      100.00

. count if ghqscale==0
    10
```

The new variable (*ln_ghq*) has a minimum value of zero because there are 15 cases in the original variable that have a value of 1 which has a logarithmic transformation value of zero. If we now graph the new variable we can see that it is closer to normal than the original variable.

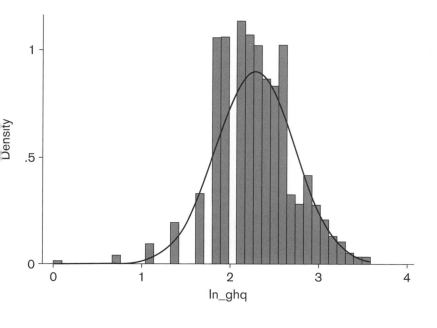

The summary statistics and test for normality produce the following output.

```
tabstat ghqscale ln_ghq, s(sk kur)
sktest ghqscale ln_ghq
```

```
. tabstat ghqscale ln_ghq, s(sk kur)

    stats |    ghqscale        ln_ghq
---------+----------------------------
 skewness |   1.364399      -.2796359
 kurtosis |   5.661401       4.491428
---------+----------------------------
```

```
. sktest ghqscale ln_ghq

              Skewness/Kurtosis tests for Normality
                                           ----- joint -----
 Variable | Pr(Skewness) Pr(Kurtosis) adj chi2(2) Prob>chi2
---------+---------------------------------------------------
 ghqscale |      0.000        0.000         .          .
   ln_ghq |      0.000        0.000         .        0.0000
```

The variable has changed from being skewed to the right to being slightly skewed to the left (from 1.36 to −0.28) and the kurtosis has moved closer to 3 so it is not so peaked. However, we have 10 extra cases without a value in the new variable, and these cases will be lost in any analysis. So, what to do about it? It could be argued that the minimum value of zero in the original variable (*ghqscale*) was done for convenience and that a score of zero does not indicate an absence of poor mental well-being. Also remember that we recoded the original 12 items to 0–3 from their survey responses that were coded 1–4 and would have made a scale with values from 12 to 48. So, one possible solution would be to shift the distribution to the right by adding 1 to everyone's score so that the variable now has values from 1 to 37. Then we use the logarithmic transformation on the new scale.

```
gen new_ghq=ghqscale+1
gen ln_ghq_2=ln(new_ghq)
su ghqscale ln_ghq ln_ghq_2
tabstat ghqscale ln_ghq ln_ghq_2, s(sk kur)
sktest ghqscale ln_ghq ln_ghq_2
```

```
. gen new_ghq=ghqscale+1
(449 missing values generated)

. gen ln_ghq_2=ln(new_ghq)
(449 missing values generated)

. su ghqscale ln_ghq ln_ghq_2

Variable |      Obs        Mean    Std. Dev.     Min          Max
---------+-----------------------------------------------------------
ghqscale |     7714    10.78727    4.945154       0           36
  ln_ghq |     7704    2.283492    .4439032       0      3.583519
ln_ghq_2 |     7714     2.38626    .4051969       0      3.610918

. tabstat ghqscale ln_ghq ln_ghq_2, s(sk kur)

   stats |   ghqscale        ln_ghq      ln_ghq_2
---------+------------------------------------------
skewness |   1.364399     -.2796359     -.2596882
kurtosis |   5.661401      4.491428      4.946262
---------------------------------------------------

. sktest ghqscale ln_ghq ln_ghq_2

            Skewness/Kurtosis tests for Normality
                                          ----- joint -----
Variable | Pr(Skewness) Pr(Kurtosis) adj chi2(2) Prob>chi2
---------+---------------------------------------------------
ghqscale |     0.000        0.000          .          .
  ln_ghq |     0.000        0.000          .       0.0000
ln_ghq_2 |     0.000        0.000          .       0.0000
```

At the start of this output you can see that Stata tells you that 449 missing values are generated in the new variable, which matches the number of cases that don't have a GHQ score in the original variable (*ghqscale*). This is checked by producing summary statistics where you can see that both the original variable (*ghqscale*) and the newly created variable (*ln_ghq_2*) have the same number of cases. The skewness and kurtosis statistics produced by the **tabstat** command indicate that the *ln_ghq_2* variable is slightly less skewed than the *ln_ghq* variable but more peaked as the kurtosis value is higher.

As with all transformations, there is a trade-off to be made between skewness and ease of interpretation. In this example we would probably use the *ghqscale* in its original form as the techniques are robust to reasonable departures from normality. The transformed GHQ score variables (either *ln_ghq* or *ln_ghq_2*) are closer to normal but the interpretation of statistics further on in this example is less intuitive. For example, a difference of means between men and women would be a difference in the logarithmic GHQ scores rather than the raw scores constructed from the items. For the rest of this demonstration we will use the untransformed *ghqscale* variable.

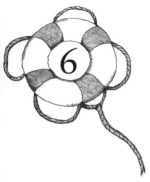

Tables and Correlations

6

In this chapter we look at some common forms of analysis: tables and correlations. We start off with two-way tables. These are sometimes called crosstabulations or crosstabs. Two-way tables are tables that use the categories of two variables to form a grid of cells. From this information, measures of association are calculated. Our explanations of the statistical tests are very brief and we focus on the basic interpretation of output. We encourage readers to consult sources that focus on the detailed explanation of these types of tests if they desire information in greater depth; for example, Agresti (2007) and Liebetrau (1983). The measures of association that you can use are largely contingent upon the level of measurement of your two variables. In Box 6.1 we present a matrix of potential measures of association by level of measurement of the two variables. The matrix is not exhaustive and other measures of association can be added as you come across them.

After two-way tables and measures of association, we move on to tables that incorporate summary statistics of variables. These can use two, three, four or even five variables in their construction.

In the section on correlations we look at parametric tests, including partial correlations and non-parametric statistics.

TWO-WAY TABLES

The **tabulate** command (shortened to **tab** or **ta**) is used with two variables to create a two-way table or crosstabulation. The level of measurement of both variables can be nominal, ordinal, or interval. While it is possible to do crosstabulations with continuous variables, the output is tedious and difficult to interpret. Furthermore, there are far more appropriate tests to use on continuous variables, as will be discussed later in Chapter 7.

Box 6.1: Matrix for appropriate tests depending on levels of measurement

'Measures of association' is a generic term for numerous statistics. There are too many to cover in this table, so five have been chosen that cover common usage. You can add measures of association to the table when you come across them.

	dichotomous	nominal	ordinal	interval
dichotomous	phi (φ)			
nominal	chi-squared (χ^2)	chi-squared (χ^2)		
ordinal	chi-squared (χ^2)	chi-squared (χ^2)	Spearman's rho (ρ)	
interval	eta (η)*	eta (η)*	Spearman's rho (ρ)	Pearson's r

* Provided the interval variable is dependent. See also differences between groups in the next chapter.

If you expect a causal association between the two variables, it is perhaps easiest to put the independent variable (i.e. the 'cause') in the columns and the dependent variable (i.e. the 'effect') in the rows. The first variable after the **tab** command makes the rows of the table while the second makes the columns. In other words, after typing **tab** (or **ta**) you would then type your dependent variable followed by your independent variable. It should be emphasized here that all the techniques described in this chapter do not assume causality. Basically what are you are testing using bivariate tests is whether there is an association – and quite literally what you should be asking when doing a crosstab is, 'Does the distribution of the values of one variable depend on the categories of another variable?' That is all crosstabulations show you – nothing more. In the case of crosstabulations using ordinal variables (described below), the question is slightly modified to, 'Is there an ordered relationship between the ordered distribution of categories?'

For ease of viewing some tables it is best to put the variable with the most categories in the rows so that the table doesn't break across the output screen. The first variable after the **tab** command will form the rows of the table and the second will form the columns. Try:

`tab sex jbstat`

and you will see that the output is divided into two parts which makes interpretation a little more difficult.

```
        |            current labour force status
   sex  | self empl in paid e unemploye retired family ca ft studen | Total
--------+----------------------------------------------------------+------
  male  |      557     2,467       374      764        15      218 | 4,599
female  |      203     2,507       161      999     1,117      180 | 5,313
--------+----------------------------------------------------------+------
 Total  |      760     4,974       535    1,763     1,132      398 | 9,912

        |          current labour force status
   sex  | long term on matern govt trng something | Total
--------+-----------------------------------------+------
  male  |      160          0        33        11 | 4,599
female  |      106         13         4        23 | 5,313
--------+-----------------------------------------+------
 Total  |      266         13        37        34 | 9,912
```

Now compare it with:

`tab jbstat sex`

shown below.

Following on with a table of sex by labour force status measured in 10 categories (*jbstat*) where sex is considered 'the cause' and job status is considered the outcome variable of interest ('the effect'):

`tab jbstat sex`

```
. ta jbstat sex

                       |          sex
  labour force status  |    male   female  |   Total
-----------------------+-------------------+--------
       self employed   |     557      203  |     760
      in paid employ   |   2,467    2,506  |   4,973
         unemployed    |     374      162  |     536
           retired     |     764      999  |   1,763
        family care    |      15    1,117  |   1,132
         ft student    |     218      180  |     398
  long term sick/disabl|     160      106  |     266
      on matern leave  |       0       13  |      13
      govt trng scheme |      33        4  |      37
      something else   |      11       23  |      34
-----------------------+-------------------+--------
               Total   |   4,599    5,313  |   9,912
```

The two-way table produced above shows the frequencies in each cell. We can see, for example, that 557 males reported being in self-employment, compared to 203 females. There were a total of 760 people who reported being self-employed. The default settings for this command also give you row and column totals. So we know that there were 4599 males and 5313 females which sums to 9912 who are included in the table calculations. You can add a variety of options to **tab**, but here we show you some of the most popular ones.

As the missing values have already been coded to missing (.), cases are not included in the table if they are missing on either of the variables. If you want to see missing values in the table then you can use the option **missing**, which can be shortened to **m**:

tab jbstat sex, m

```
. ta jbstat sex, m
```

labour force status	sex male	female	Total
self employed	557	203	760
in paid employ	2,467	2,506	4,973
unemployed	374	162	536
retired	764	999	1,763
family care	15	1,117	1,132
ft student	218	180	398
long term sick/disabl	160	106	266
on matern leave	0	13	13
govt trng scheme	33	4	37
something else	11	23	34
.	234	118	352
Total	4,833	5,431	10,264

You can see from this table that there are no cases with missing values on *sex* but 352 cases with missing values on *jbstat* as shown by the row category with a dot (.); 234 males and 118 females.

Measures of association are available with the option **all**. They will tell you if the results reported in your table are statistically significant. In other words, how likely is it that the results are due to chance alone, or how likely is it that they represent true associations in the population? Pearson's chi-squared, likelihood-ratio chi-squared, Cramér's V, gamma, and Kendall's tau-b are reported.

As with most software, Stata will compute the statistics but you have to make the decision about which statistics are the most appropriate. In the example below Stata will produce tau-b and gamma statistics, but these are not appropriate for this table.

tab jbstat sex, all

```
. ta jbstat sex, all

                       |        sex
   labour force status |    male   female |    Total
-----------------------+------------------+--------
         self employed |     557      203 |      760
       in paid employ |   2,467    2,506 |    4,973
           unemployed |     374      162 |      536
              retired |     764      999 |    1,763
          family care |      15    1,117 |    1,132
           ft student |     218      180 |      398
  long term sick/disabl |    160      106 |      266
       on matern leave |       0       13 |       13
      govt trng scheme |      33        4 |       37
       something else |      11       23 |       34
-----------------------+------------------+--------
                Total |   4,599    5,313 |    9,912

         Pearson chi2(9) =  1.4e+03    Pr  =  0.000
likelihood-ratio chi2(9) =  1.7e+03    Pr  =  0.000
             Cramér's V =  0.3709
                  gamma =  0.3142    ASE  =  0.015
        Kendall's tau-b =  0.1879    ASE  =  0.009
```

The first two measures of association – Pearson's and likelihood ratio chi-squared – are shown with their p value (i.e. their likelihood that the results are due to chance alone). A general guideline is that you would be looking for these values to be less than 0.05 in order to consider them statistically significant, although other common values are 0.01 and 0.001. These values should be determined a priori (before conducting the tests!). You will also notice that there is a number in parentheses after chi2. This is the degrees of freedom associated with the statistical test. If you look at a table for the chi-square distribution (which is at the back of most statistics textbooks), you would look for 9 degrees of freedom and a 0.95 level of significance. You would find a value of 16.92. The chi-square statistic reported is in excess of 1000 (which is a lot bigger than 16.92!) and therefore you can reject the null hypothesis that the distribution of one of the variables did not depend on the categories of another. The p value is a shortcut to this information (rejecting the null). In other words, both pieces of information lead to the same conclusion.

It is useful to briefly explain the other measures of association. Cramér's V statistic is reported on its own (it ranges from 0 to 1, with 1 indicating a perfect relationship) and is relevant here because both variables are nominal. The value reported is 0.3710, which is considered strong (generally values around 0.25 are considered strong; see Liebetrau 1983). Although not relevant to the current example as both variables used in the crosstabulation are nominal, gamma and Kendall's tau-b range between −1 and +1 and are reported with their asymptotic standard error (ASE), which is a type of standard error that can be used for statistical significance tests (i.e. in place of p).

If you just want one of the measures of association use **chi2** for Pearson's chi-squared, **lrchi2** for likelihood-ratio chi-squared, **gamma** for gamma, **v** for Cramér's V, and **taub** for Kendall's tau-b.

The statistic for Fisher's exact test (typically used for 2 × 2 tables) can be obtained with the option **exact**. An example would be if we created a table of a dichotomous measure of being married (1 = married, 0 = not married) with sex.

tab married sex, exact

```
. ta married sex, exact

    married |        sex
  indicator |    male    female |    Total
------------+--------------------+---------
not married |   1,886     2,369 |    4,255
    married |   2,947     3,062 |    6,009
------------+--------------------+---------
      Total |   4,833     5,431 |   10,264

          Fisher's exact =  0.000
  1-sided Fisher's exact =  0.000
```

We can see that the *p* value is 0.000, which is less than the standard *p* value of 0.05, so we can conclude that the distribution in the table is unlikely to be due to chance alone. The one-sided Fisher's exact test is used if you have a directional hypothesis – for instance, if you had a reason to believe the females were more likely to be married than males, rather than a two-tailed test, which just hypothesizes that there will be some kind of difference in the distribution of the cases in the table by sex. Typically it is about half the size of the Fisher's exact test, although in our example the *p* value is so small that dividing it by 2 still produces 0.000.

Percentages can be included in the table cells by using options. If you are interested in including row percentages in your crosstabulation, use the **row** option after the **tab** command. The following examples use the variables self-reported health status (*hlstat*) and *sex*.

tab hlstat sex, row

```
. tab hlstat sex, row

  ----------------+
    Key           |
  ----------------|
    frequency     |
   row percentage |
  ----------------+

  health over |        sex
last 12 months |   male    female  |     Total
---------------+--------------------+----------
     excellent |  1,536     1,394   |    2,930
               |  52.42     47.58   |   100.00
---------------+--------------------+----------
          good |  2,149     2,464   |    4,613
               |  46.59     53.41   |   100.00
---------------+--------------------+----------
          fair |    808     1,045   |    1,853
               |  43.60     56.40   |   100.00
---------------+--------------------+----------
          poor |    246       395   |      641
               |  38.38     61.62   |   100.00
---------------+--------------------+----------
     very poor |     93       126   |      219
               |  42.47     57.53   |   100.00
---------------+--------------------+----------
         Total |  4,832     5,424   |   10,256
               |  47.11     52.89   |   100.00
```

You can now see that of all the individuals who reported excellent health, 52.42% were males and 47.58% were females. Similarly if you are interested in column percentages you would type **column** or **col**

tab hlstat sex, col

```
. tab hlstat sex, col

+------------------+
| Key              |
|------------------|
|     frequency    |
| column percentage|
+------------------+

   health over |         sex
last 12 months |    male   female |     Total
---------------+------------------+----------
     excellent |   1,536    1,394 |     2,930
               |   31.79    25.70 |     28.57
---------------+------------------+----------
          good |   2,149    2,464 |     4,613
               |   44.47    45.43 |     44.98
---------------+------------------+----------
          fair |     808    1,045 |     1,853
               |   16.72    19.27 |     18.07
---------------+------------------+----------
          poor |     246      395 |       641
               |    5.09     7.28 |      6.25
---------------+------------------+----------
     very poor |      93      126 |       219
               |    1.92     2.32 |      2.14
---------------+------------------+----------
         Total |   4,832    5,424 |    10,256
               |  100.00   100.00 |    100.00
```

The column percentages tell you that of out of all males, 31.79% reported having excellent health compared to 25.70% of all females.

The option **cell** tells Stata to produce cell percentages when the total of the cell percentages equals 100%.

tab hlstat sex, cell

```
. tab hlstat sex, cell

+------------------+
| Key              |
|------------------|
|     frequency    |
| cell percentage  |
+------------------+
```

health over last 12 months	sex male	female	Total
excellent	1,536	1,394	2,930
	14.98	13.59	28.57
good	2,149	2,464	4,613
	20.95	24.02	44.98
fair	808	1,045	1,853
	7.88	10.19	18.07
poor	246	395	641
	2.40	3.85	6.25
very poor	93	126	219
	0.91	1.23	2.14
Total	4,832	5,424	10,256
	47.11	52.89	100.00

In this table the marginals – the right-hand column and the bottom row – add up to 100% while all the cells 'inside' the table also add up to 100%, so, for example, males who report their health as 'good' (N = 2149) are 20.95% of the whole sample N = 10,256).

You can see in the three examples above that Stata gives you a key to the cell contents which becomes more useful if you combine options. You can combine options to give you the exact table you need. For example, if we wish to have column and cell percentages along with Pearson's chi-squared and likelihood ratio chi-squared statistics:

`tab hlstat sex, col cell chi2 lr`

. tab hlstat sex, col cell chi lr

```
+------------------+
| Key              |
|------------------|
|      frequency   |
| column percentage |
|  cell percentage |
+------------------+
```

health over last 12 months	sex male	female	Total
excellent	1,536	1,394	2,930
	31.79	25.70	28.57
	14.98	13.59	28.57
good	2,149	2,464	4,613
	44.47	45.43	44.98
	20.95	24.02	44.98
fair	808	1,045	1,853
	16.72	19.27	18.07
	7.88	10.19	18.07
poor	246	395	641
	5.09	7.28	6.25
	2.40	3.85	6.25
very poor	93	126	219
	1.92	2.32	2.14
	0.91	1.23	2.14
Total	4,832	5,424	10,256
	100.00	100.00	100.00
	47.11	52.89	100.00

$$\text{Pearson chi2}(4) = 64.3546 \quad Pr = 0.000$$
$$\text{likelihood-ratio chi2}(4) = 64.5617 \quad Pr = 0.000$$

If you prefer to copy and paste your tables into Excel for graphing, a useful option is **nofreq**. This tells Stata not to report

the cell or marginal frequencies. It must be combined with another
option, otherwise no output is shown. In our example we wish to
see column percentages so we add the **col** option.

tab hlstat sex, nofreq col

```
. tab hlstat sex, nofreq col

   health over |         sex
 last 12 months |    male   female  |     Total
----------------+-------------------+----------
      excellent |   31.79    25.70  |     28.57
           good |   44.47    45.43  |     44.98
           fair |   16.72    19.27  |     18.07
           poor |    5.09     7.28  |      6.25
      very poor |    1.92     2.32  |      2.14
----------------+-------------------+----------
          Total |  100.00   100.00  |    100.00
```

Note that as only one piece of information per cell has been
requested that a table key is not shown. The table key can be suppressed by using the **nokey** option, but we suggest leaving it
shown until you become familiar with the way Stata presents
its output.

The **nofreq** option is also useful if you are only interested in
the measures of association being reported rather than whole
tables. You just type **nofreq** followed by the measure(s) of association you are interested to see. In the example below, we select
only Pearson's chi-squared statistic.

tab hlstat sex, nofreq chi2

```
. tab hlstat sex, nofreq chi2
         Pearson chi2(4) =   64.3546   Pr = 0.000
```

CONDITIONAL CROSSTABULATIONS

In combination with the **bysort** command from Chapter 4, you
can use the **tabulate** command to do conditional crosstabulations. For example, if you wanted to see crosstabulations of self-
reported health (*hlstat*) by registered disabled status (*hldsbl*) for
both sexes:

bysort sex: ta hlstat hldsbl

All the options of the **ta** command are still available when you separate your results using a **bysort** command, so in this example we also want each table to have column percentages along with Pearson's chi-squared statistic:

bysort sex: ta hlstat hldsbl, col chi2

```
. bysort sex: ta hlstat hldsbl, col chi2

-------------------------------------------------------
-> sex = male

+-------------------+
| Key               |
|-------------------|
|      frequency    |
| column percentage |
+-------------------+

    health over | registered disabled
last 12 months |       yes        no |     Total
---------------+--------------------+---------
     excellent |        10     1,519 |     1,529
               |      4.12     33.20 |     31.74
---------------+--------------------+---------
          good |        56     2,088 |     2,144
               |     23.05     45.64 |     44.50
---------------+--------------------+---------
          fair |        65       742 |       807
               |     26.75     16.22 |     16.75
---------------+--------------------+---------
          poor |        70       176 |       246
               |     28.81      3.85 |      5.11
---------------+--------------------+---------
     very poor |        42        50 |        92
               |     17.28      1.09 |      1.91
---------------+--------------------+---------
         Total |       243     4,575 |     4,818
               |    100.00    100.00 |    100.00

       Pearson chi2(4) = 701.5820   Pr = 0.000
```

```
-------------------------------------------------
-> sex = female

+-------------------+
| Key               |
|-------------------|
|      frequency    |
| column percentage |
+-------------------+

  health over | registered disabled
last 12 months |     yes        no |    Total
---------------+-------------------+---------
     excellent |       3     1,387 |    1,390
               |    1.59     26.62 |    25.74
---------------+-------------------+---------
          good |      39     2,413 |    2,452
               |   20.63     46.31 |    45.41
---------------+-------------------+---------
          fair |      60       978 |    1,038
               |   31.75     18.77 |    19.22
---------------+-------------------+---------
          poor |      55       339 |      394
               |   29.10      6.51 |     7.30
---------------+-------------------+---------
     very poor |      32        94 |      126
               |   16.93      1.80 |     2.33
---------------+-------------------+---------
         Total |     189     5,211 |    5,400
               |  100.00    100.00 |   100.00

   Pearson chi2(4) = 393.3277   Pr = 0.000
```

You can see that the tables for self-reported health status and registered disabled are reported first for males and then for females. You can see that the chi-squared statistic was statistically significant for both groups with p values of 0.000.

You can also refine your analysis by using an **if** statement. The **if** statement tells Stata the condition(s) that you want to set. So, if you wanted to do a table of health status by sex but only for people who are in some age range, say between 20 and 30, you would use an **if** statement after the **ta** command. We set the age

range to be between 20 and 30 by specifying that cases where the
age is greater than 19 and less than 31 should be included in the
analysis.

ta hlstat sex if (age>19 & age<31),all

```
. ta hlstat sex if (age>19 & age<31),all

    health over |          sex
last 12 months |    male    female |     Total
---------------+-------------------+---------
     excellent |     412       338 |       750
          good |     447       548 |       995
          fair |     135       201 |       336
          poor |      33        65 |        98
     very poor |       5        11 |        16
---------------+-------------------+---------
         Total |   1,032     1,163 |     2,195

         Pearson chi2(4) =  35.5252   Pr = 0.000
likelihood-ratio chi2(4) =  35.7583   Pr = 0.000
             Cramér's V =    0.1272
                  gamma =    0.2060   ASE = 0.034
        Kendall's tau-b =    0.1180   ASE = 0.020
```

Notice that the **all** option goes after the **if** statement and that a
space after the comma is not necessary.

Of course, you could take this a step even further. You could
use the **bysort** command in combination with an **if** statement
to further refine the tables. For example:

**bysort sex: ta hlstat hldsbl if (age>59 & ///
    age<81),col chi2**

This would generate two crosstabulations, one for men and one
for women, of self-reported health by registered disabled status
for persons aged 60–80. The tables would contain column per
centages and report Pearson's chi-squared statistic.

```
. bysort sex: ta hlstat hldsbl if (age>59 & ///
    age<81),col chi2
```

```
---------------------------------------------------------
-> sex = male

+-------------------+
| Key               |
|-------------------|
|      frequency    |
| column percentage |
+-------------------+

  health over | registered disabled
last 12 months |     yes        no  |    Total
---------------+--------------------+---------
   excellent  |       5       209  |      214
             |    4.24     25.49  |    22.81
---------------+--------------------+---------
       good  |      25       354  |      379
             |   21.19     43.17  |    40.41
---------------+--------------------+---------
       fair  |      32       195  |      227
             |   27.12     23.78  |    24.20
---------------+--------------------+---------
       poor  |      36        51  |       87
             |   30.51      6.22  |     9.28
---------------+--------------------+---------
  very poor  |      20        11  |       31
             |   16.95      1.34  |     3.30
---------------+--------------------+---------
      Total  |     118       820  |      938
             |  100.00    100.00  |   100.00

    Pearson chi2(4) = 174.8807   Pr = 0.000

---------------------------------------------------------
-> sex = female

+-------------------+
| Key               |
|-------------------|
|      frequency    |
| column percentage |
+-------------------+
```

```
  health over | registered disabled
last 12 months |      yes        no |    Total
---------------+--------------------+---------
     excellent |        0       210 |      210
               |     0.00     18.88 |    17.50
---------------+--------------------+---------
          good |       16       494 |      510
               |    18.18     44.42 |    42.50
---------------+--------------------+---------
          fair |       31       275 |      306
               |    35.23     24.73 |    25.50
---------------+--------------------+---------
          poor |       28        92 |      120
               |    31.82      8.27 |    10.00
---------------+--------------------+---------
     very poor |       13        41 |       54
               |    14.77      3.69 |     4.50
---------------+--------------------+---------
         Total |       88     1,112 |    1,200
               |   100.00    100.00 |   100.00
```

Pearson chi2(4) = 100.8323   Pr = 0.000

To produce two-way tables using pull-down menus, see Box 6.2.

Box 6.2: Crosstabulations using pull-down menus

To obtain crosstabulations or two-way tables by using the pull-down menus use the following path:

Statistics → Summaries, tables, and tests → Tables → Two-way tables with measures of association

This takes you to the **tabulate2 – Two-way tables** dialogue box and its **Main** tab shown below. The row and column variables are entered by typing in or scrolling down. All the other options for crosstabulations (test statistics and cell contents) are then ticked if they are required.

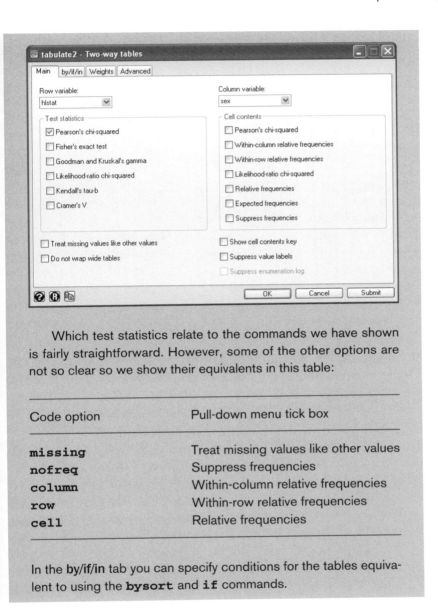

Which test statistics relate to the commands we have shown is fairly straightforward. However, some of the other options are not so clear so we show their equivalents in this table:

Code option	Pull-down menu tick box
`missing`	Treat missing values like other values
`nofreq`	Suppress frequencies
`column`	Within-column relative frequencies
`row`	Within-row relative frequencies
`cell`	Relative frequencies

In the **by/if/in** tab you can specify conditions for the tables equivalent to using the **bysort** and **if** commands.

MULTIPLE TWO-WAY TABLES

The command **tab2** will produce two-way tables between all variables in a variable list. For example, the command

```
tab2 hlstat sex married
```

will produce two-way tables for all three variables with one another. So there will be a table for *hlstat* by *sex*, *hlstat* by *married*, and *sex* by *married*. All possible two-way tables (i.e. pair combinations) will be produced, depending on the number of variables specified. For three variables, there are 3 possible combinations, for four variables there would be 6, and so on.

```
. tab2 hlstat sex married

-> tabulation of hlstat by sex

   health over |          sex
 last 12 months |    male     female |    Total
----------------+--------------------+---------
      excellent |   1,536      1,394 |    2,930
           good |   2,149      2,464 |    4,613
           fair |     808      1,045 |    1,853
           poor |     246        395 |      641
      very poor |      93        126 |      219
----------------+--------------------+---------
          Total |   4,832      5,424 |   10,256

-> tabulation of hlstat by married

   health over |   married indicator
 last 12 months |  not marri   married |    Total
----------------+--------------------+---------
      excellent |   1,187      1,743 |    2,930
           good |   1,870      2,743 |    4,613
           fair |     807      1,046 |    1,853
           poor |     283        358 |      641
      very poor |     102        117 |      219
----------------+--------------------+---------
          Total |   4,249      6,007 |   10,256

-> tabulation of sex by married

                |   married indicator
            sex |  not marri   married |    Total
----------------+--------------------+-------
           male |   1,886      2,947 |    4,833
         female |   2,369      3,062 |    5,431
----------------+--------------------+-------
          Total |   4,255      6,009 |   10,264
```

The **tab2** command can be combined with **bysort** and **if** in the same way as the **tab** command.

To create multiple two-way tables using pull-down menus, see Box 6.3.

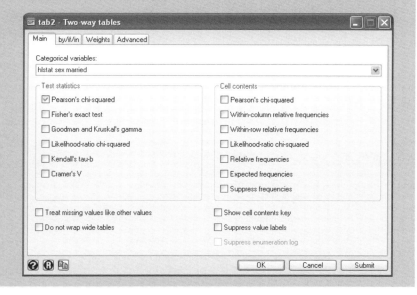

Box 6.3: Multiple crosstabulations using pull-down menus

The pull-down menu equivalent of the **tab2** command is found at:

Statistics → Summaries, tables, and tests → Tables → All possible two-way tabulations

This takes you to the **tab2 – Two-way tables** dialogue box where you enter the list of variables by either typing or scrolling down and selecting by right-clicking on all the variables you want including in the list. All of the options are the same as the single two-way table window shown in Box 6.2.

COMBINING TABLES AND SUMMARY STATISTICS

You can use **su** as an option within a **tabulate** command to produce tables that report means and standard deviations for an interval variable across categories of a nominal or ordinal variable.

For example, if you wanted to see the mean ages of people according to their marital status you could use any of the following three commands.

The first command is a simple **ta** which uses **su** as an option in order to report the means of a second variable.

ta mastat, su(age)

```
. ta mastat, su(age)
        marital |            Summary of age
         status |        Mean    Std. Dev.      Freq.
  --------------+-----------------------------------
        married |   47.198536    14.944372        6009
      living as |   32.378338    12.135964         674
        widowed |   72.182448    11.085019         866
       divorced |   46.919355     12.65734         434
      separated |   42.444444    14.628133         189
      never mar |   28.999044    15.932846        2092
  --------------+-----------------------------------
          Total |   44.524552    18.467111       10264
```

By default the means, standard deviations and frequencies are reported. This may be more information than you need. If you want a simpler table that just reports means (and not standard deviations and frequencies), you would use **means** as a option:

ta mastat sex, su(age) means

```
. ta mastat, su(age) means
                | Summary of
        marital |     age
         status |       Mean
  --------------+------------
        married |   47.198536
      living as |   32.378338
        widowed |   72.182448
       divorced |   46.919355
      separated |   42.444444
      never mar |   28.999044
  --------------+------------
          Total |   44.524552
```

The next command uses **su** in combination with **bysort**. The output here differs from the previous example as summary statistics are presented separately for all marital status groups. Unlike the example above, the minimum and maximum values are also reported.

bysort mastat: su age

```
. bysort mastat: su age

----------------------------------------------------------
-> mastat = married
    Variable |     Obs       Mean   Std. Dev.   Min   Max
-------------+--------------------------------------------
         age |    6009   47.19854    14.94437    18    94

----------------------------------------------------------
-> mastat = living a
    Variable |     Obs       Mean   Std. Dev.   Min   Max
-------------+--------------------------------------------
         age |     674   32.37834    12.13596    17    91

----------------------------------------------------------
-> mastat = widowed
    Variable |     Obs       Mean   Std. Dev.   Min   Max
-------------+--------------------------------------------
         age |     866   72.18245    11.08502    27    96

----------------------------------------------------------
-> mastat = divorced
    Variable |     Obs       Mean   Std. Dev.   Min   Max
-------------+--------------------------------------------
         age |     434   46.91935    12.65734    22    85

----------------------------------------------------------
-> mastat = separate
    Variable |     Obs       Mean   Std. Dev.   Min   Max
-------------+--------------------------------------------
         age |     189   42.44444    14.62813    22    86

----------------------------------------------------------
-> mastat = never ma
    Variable |     Obs       Mean   Std. Dev.   Min   Max
-------------+--------------------------------------------
         age |    2092   28.99904    15.93285    16    97
```

As we've said before, there is often more than one way to get to essentially the same results. Another command that can produce similar types of tables for you is **tabstat**. You can get very similar results to the ones produced above with the following command:

tabstat age, by(mastat)

```
. tabstat age, by(mastat)

Summary for variables: age
      by categories of: mastat (marital status)

            mastat |       mean
-------------------+-----------
           married |   47.19854
  living as couple |   32.37834
           widowed |   72.18245
          divorced |   46.91935
         separated |   42.44444
     never married |   28.99904
-------------------+-----------
             Total |   44.52455
-------------------------------
```

The command **tabstat** is for creating tables of summary statistics, typically for variables at the interval level (i.e. because the means, standard deviations, etc. for nominal and ordinal variables don't mean much). You can condition the results produced in the table by another variable, like we did above – we asked for the means of age conditioned on marital status. In this sense, **tabstat** is like the **ta** command combined with the option **su**. It is different in that you can request more types of statistics to be presented. For example, you can request the inter-quartile range (**iqr**), kurtosis (**k**), skewness (**ske**), variance (**v**) and coefficient of variation (**cv**), as well as others. See **help tabstat** for a full list of options.

For example, you could have Stata report means, minimum values and the 25th percentile using the following command:

tabstat age, by(mastat) stats(mean min p25)

```
. tabstat age, by(mastat) stats(mean min p25)

Summary for variables: age
      by categories of: mastat (marital status)

        mastat |        mean     min     p25
---------------+------------------------------
       married |    47.19854      18      35
living as couple |  32.37834      17      24
       widowed |    72.18245      27      67
      divorced |    46.91935      22      37
     separated |    42.44444      22      31
 never married |    28.99904      16      19
---------------+------------------------------
         Total |    44.52455      16      29
-----------------------------------------------
```

The command **tabstat** also has the advantage of allowing you to customize the presentation of the table. For example, by using the command

tabstat age, by(mastat) s(mean range iqr) ///
   nototal

we can request that the mean, range, and inter-quartile range are reported, and the **nototal** option tells Stata not to report a final line with column totals.

```
. tabstat age, by(mastat) s(mean range iqr) ///
    nototal

Summary for variables: age
      by categories of: mastat (marital status)

        mastat |        mean   range     iqr
---------------+------------------------------
       married |    47.19854      76      23
living as couple |  32.37834      74      13
       widowed |    72.18245      69      13
      divorced |    46.91935      63      19
     separated |    42.44444      64      20
 never married |    28.99904      81      13
-----------------------------------------------
```

We can also use the **col(var)** option to display the variables in the columns of the tables instead of the statistics, which is the default.

```
. tabstat age, by(mastat) stats(mean range ///
    iqr) col(var) nototal
```

Summary statistics: mean, range, iqr
  by categories of: mastat (marital status)

```
          mastat |         age
-----------------+-----------
         married |   47.19854
                 |         76
                 |         23
-----------------+-----------
living as couple |   32.37834
                 |         74
                 |         13
-----------------+-----------
         widowed |   72.18245
                 |         69
                 |         13
-----------------+-----------
        divorced |   46.91935
                 |         63
                 |         19
-----------------+-----------
       separated |   42.44444
                 |         64
                 |         20
-----------------+-----------
   never married |   28.99904
                 |         81
                 |         13
-----------------------------
```

To create tables of summary statistics using pull-down menus, see Box 6.4.

Box 6.4: Tables of summary statistics

The pull-down menu equivalent of the **tab** command with the **su** option is found at:

Statistics → Summaries, tables, and tests → Tables → One/two-way table of summary statistics

This brings you to the **Main** tab in the **tabsum – One/two-way table of summary statistics** dialogue box. This will also make one-way tables with summary statistics of a second variable. Either type in or scroll down and select the two variables for the categories of the table. The variable being summarized in the cells is entered in the **Summarize variable** box. There are options to customize the output. The default is for means, standard deviations and frequencies to be reported but each of these can be suppressed with the tick boxes. In the **by/if/in** tab you can specify conditions for the tables equivalent to using **bysort** and **if**. In this example we have used the variable *mastat* to form the rows of the table (**Variable 1** box) and *sex* to form the columns (**Variable 2** box) with the mean of the *age* variable reported in each cell. The standard deviations, frequencies and number of observations are all suppressed using the tick boxes.

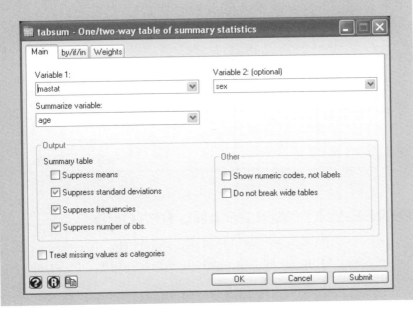

▶   The pull-down menu equivalent of the `tabstat` command is found at:

Statistics → Summaries, tables, and tests → Tables → Table of summary statistics (tabstat)

This brings you to the **Main** tab in the **tabstat – Tables of summary statistics** dialogue box where you specify which variables you want summarized in the **Variables** box. The categorical variable to form the table is specified in the **Group statistics by variable** box. If this isn't specified then the summary statistics refer to the whole sample in the open data set. In this example we want to create a table of categories of the *mastat* variable that shows the mean of the variables *age* and *ghqscale* for each category. As with all the other tabulation commands, you can specify conditions for the tables equivalent to using `bysort` and `if` in the **by/if/in** tab.

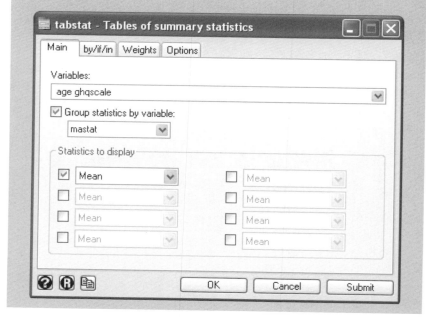

THREE-WAY TABLES AND BEYOND

A natural extension of the two-way table is the three-way table. A three-way table gives you more information by tabulating two variables with each other with the mean of a third variable reported in the cells. This can be achieved with the generic command `ta variable1 variable2, su(variable3)`

so you would end up with a table of *variable1* by *variable2*, but instead of the frequencies of each cell, you would have the mean value of *variable3* reported.

It makes more sense to use an example. Suppose we are interested in knowing the mean age of men and women by marital status. We can get this with the command:

`ta mastat sex, su(age)`

```
. ta mastat sex, su(age)
            Means, Standard Deviations and
                Frequencies of age
```

marital status	sex male	female	Total
married	48.603325 15.081306 2947	45.846506 14.687464 3062	47.198536 14.944372 6009
living as	33.458084 12.36032 334	31.317647 11.833866 340	32.378338 12.135964 674
widowed	73.704142 10.53543 169	71.813486 11.190343 697	72.182448 11.085019 866
divorced	47.886667 12.970559 150	46.408451 12.481593 284	46.919355 12.65734 434
separated	44.915254 14.152236 59	41.323077 14.756008 130	42.444444 14.628133 189
never mar	28.035775 14.262205 1174	30.230937 17.775071 918	28.999044 15.932846 2092
Total	43.370991 17.986082 4833	45.551096 18.827175 5431	44.524552 18.467111 10264

We can see here that the average age of a married man in this sample is 48.60 years, with a standard deviation of 15.08, while the average age of a married female is 45.85 with a standard deviation of 14.69. The overall average age of married people is 47.20 years, as indicated in the row total, while the overall average age of men in the sample is 43.37, and 45.55 years for females, as indicated in the column totals. If you did not want the standard deviations and frequencies which come with the default settings you can specify a **means** option:

ta mastat sex, su(age) means

```
. ta mastat sex, su(age) means

                         Means of age
        marital |              sex
         status |       male      female |        Total
   -------------+------------------------+------------
        married |   48.603325   45.846506 |   47.198536
      living as |   33.458084   31.317647 |   32.378338
        widowed |   73.704142   71.813486 |   72.182448
       divorced |   47.886667   46.408451 |   46.919355
      separated |   44.915254   41.323077 |   42.444444
      never mar |   28.035775   30.230937 |   28.999044
   -------------+------------------------+------------
          Total |   43.370991   45.551096 |   44.524552
```

These ways of creating three-way tables using the **ta** command are also available for **tab2**, so, for example, the command below would create three two-way tables each with the mean age in the cells.

tab2 hlstat sex married, su(age) means

The **table** command in Stata is useful for producing customized tables, particularly three-way tables. Look at the results for:

table mastat sex, c(m age)

```
. table mastat sex, c(m age)
```

```
                      |          sex
   marital status     |     male       female
----------------------+----------------------
          married     |   48.6033     45.8465
 living as couple     |   33.4581     31.3176
          widowed     |   73.7041     71.8135
         divorced     |   47.8867     46.4085
        separated     |   44.9153     41.3231
    never married     |   28.0358     30.2309
```

Note that the **c** in the command means content of the cells and the **m** indicates that the mean value of the *age* variable should be displayed. As with other tabulation commands, there is a variety of options for reported statistics and presentation. For example, we use the **table** command to also include the median (**med**) of the *ghqscale* variable in the cells and format (**f**) the cells to reduce the number of decimal places shown. The **table** command is the most flexible way of presenting results such as these.

table mastat sex, c(m age med ghqscale) ///
   f(%4.2f)

```
. table mastat sex, c(m age med ghqscale) ///
    f(%4.2f)

                      |          sex
   marital status     |     male       female
----------------------+----------------------
          married     |    48.60        45.85
                      |     9.00        10.00
 living as couple     |    33.46        31.32
                      |     9.00        10.00
          widowed     |    73.70        71.81
                      |    10.00        11.00
         divorced     |    47.89        46.41
                      |    10.00        12.00
        separated     |    44.92        41.32
                      |    11.00        12.00
    never married     |    28.04        30.23
                      |     9.00        10.00
```

The **table** command has ability to create 'four-way' and 'five-way' tables as well (see Box 6.5), with various customizing options for statistics and presentation. For example, the command

table jbstat married sex, c(m age)

will produce a table for labour force status (*jbstat*) by *married* and *sex*, with the mean values of *age* reported in the cells.

```
. table jbstat married sex, c(m age)

---------------------------------------------------------------------
                        |          sex and married indicator
                        |   ------ male ------   ----- female ------
 labour force status    | not married  married  not married  married
------------------------+--------------------------------------------
        self employed   |   38.1635   44.9221     40.0877   43.4795
      in paid employ    |   29.9297   42.2769     32.2243   41.1005
          unemployed    |   30.848    42.9353     29.6754   37.2917
             retired    |   74.3148   70.5821     73.1495   67.0911
         family care    |   36.4      44.9        51.1145   44.5823
          ft student    |   18.8545   35.6        19.4226   34.3333
long term sick/disabled |   50.25     53.8462     52.3276   50.5208
      on matern leave   |                              20   29.8333
      govt trng scheme  |   21.1538   37               29
      something else    |   27.1429   43.25        54.3     41.3077
---------------------------------------------------------------------
```

Some of the cells are blank, such as males who were on maternity leave, as there were no observations. You should note that the variable with the most categories should be specified first – in this case *jbstat* – so that the table is easier to read. You can use nominal and ordinal variables for these tables (just the one variable you want the mean value reported for must be interval), but the more categories you have, the more complicated your table is going to be. This is why we have displayed the simpler *married* variable rather than the original variable *mastat*.

The final message before moving on to correlations is that there are a lot of different ways to make two- and three-way tables in Stata. You will find the command that you like the best, after practising with the ones we have shown you. There are special options available in the different commands, but the basics are pretty much the same. You just have to figure out the commands that are most suited for the types of results you are interested in presenting.

Box 6.5: Three-way and higher-way tables using pull-down menus

The pull-down menu equivalent of the **table** command is found at:

Statistics → **Summaries, tables, and tests** → **Tables** → **Table of summary statistics (table)**

This brings you to the **Main** tab in the **table - Tables of summary statistics** dialogue box. Here you specify your row and column variables; in this example we have used the variables *jbstat* and *smoker*, respectively. If you wish you can also specify **Superrow** and **Supercolumn** variables; for illustration of how complex the tables can be we have chosen *sex* and *married*. The cell contents are specified by the numbered rows of boxes; we have chosen the mean of *age*, but up to five statistics could be specified from different variables if needed.

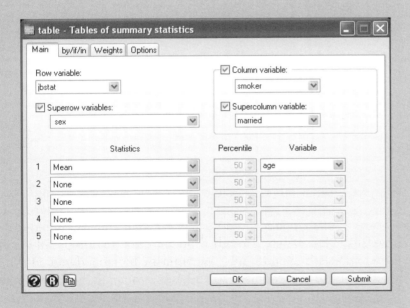

This will produce the following table – quite a bit of information! And you could further combine this with **bysort** or **if** in the **by/if/in** tab. ▶

▶

```
--------------------------------------------------------------
                        | married indicator and smoker
 sex and labour force   | - not marr -    -- married --
              status    |   yes      no      yes      no
------------------------+-------------------------------------
male                    |
        self employed   | 34.85    40.06    41.87    46.16
       in paid employ   | 29.99    29.93    41.80    42.43
          unemployed    | 29.95    31.99    39.12    46.49
             retired    | 71.81    75.26    68.57    71.07
         family care    | 37.25    33.00    49.00    40.80
          ft student    | 19.05    18.81       .     35.60
long term sick/disabled | 50.32    50.16    52.64    54.84
      on matern leave   |    .        .        .        .
      govt trng scheme  | 24.75    19.56    32.00    39.00
       something else   | 26.25    28.33    36.00    45.67
------------------------+-------------------------------------
female                  |
        self employed   | 38.50    40.82    42.24    43.90
       in paid employ   | 32.65    32.01    41.16    41.08
          unemployed    | 29.04    29.89    38.50    36.43
             retired    | 69.86    74.00    66.19    67.26
         family care    | 36.04    60.57    42.11    45.52
          ft student    | 19.77    19.34    36.00    34.18
long term sick/disabled | 50.21    54.45    49.11    51.37
      on matern leave   |    .     20.00    30.00    29.80
      govt trng scheme  |    .     29.00       .        .
       something else   | 39.33    60.71    41.67    41.20
--------------------------------------------------------------
```

The **Options** tab gives you a number of ways of customizing the presentation of your table. In this example we have used the format option so that the figures are presented concisely (there are numerous formats to use – we suggest experimenting to find out which works best for you) and also specified that the missing statistics are shown with a dot (.) rather than left blank, which is the default.

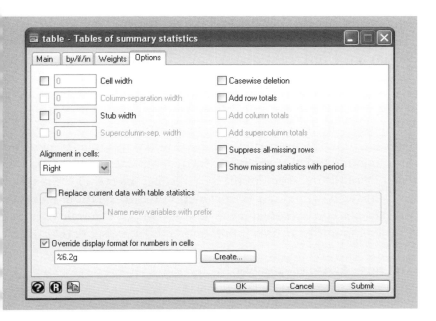

CORRELATIONS

There are two types of correlations that are widely used in the social and behavioural sciences – Pearson's product-moment correlation and the non-parametric varieties which include Spearman's rank correlation coefficient and Kendall's rank-order correlation coefficient. The most important thing to remember is that all statistics have their own set of assumptions – that is, the conditions under which they work properly. Pearson's product-moment correlation measures the linear association between two variables and both variables must be measured at the interval level. Like most non-parametric statistics, the big difference between this type of estimate and its parametric cousin is that non-parametric statistics are calculated based on ranks while parametric statistics focus on mean values. As we know, means are 'meaningless' unless we have variables measured at the interval level. Thus, we typically use Spearman's or Kendall's calculation when we have ordinal variables.

Pearson's product-moment correlation

The command **correlate** (which can be shortened to **corr** or **cor**) is used to create Pearson's product-moment correlations between variables (usually just referred to as Pearson's r). If you type **cor** followed by a list of variables you will get a correlation matrix for all those variables. Observations are excluded from the calculation due to missing values on a listwise basis. This means that cases must be present on all items in the variable list in order to be included in the analysis. If a respondent failed to answer even one of the questions in the variable list, the rest of the respondent's answers would not be included in the correlation. Here we correlate the three interval level variables in our example data set: age (*age*), monthly income (*fimn*) and GHQ scale score (*ghqscale*).

cor age fimn ghqscale

```
. cor age fimn ghqscale
(obs=9613)

             |      age      fimn   ghqscale
-------------+------------------------------
     age |   1.0000
    fimn |  -0.0890    1.0000
     ghq |   0.0511   -0.0892     1.0000
```

Across the diagonal are the variables correlated with themselves, which is always a perfect correlation (i.e. 1.00). Pearson's correlation values range from −1.0 to 1.0, with values closer to +1 or −1 indicating a stronger association. A correlation of 0 means there is no linear association. A positive association means there is a tendency for the values of one variable to increase as the values of the other variables increase. This also holds true if the values decrease – as one decreases, the other decreases as well. A negative relationship means that as one variable increases, the other decreases, and vice versa (i.e. as one variable decreases, the other increases). Remember, correlations do not imply causation; that they simply tell you the extent to which variables tend to increase or decrease together. This relationship does not tell you that one variable causes the other to change – only that there is some association between their values. In terms of interpretation, values below 0.30 suggest there is little association between the variables (see Hinkle et al. 1988).

You can also specify that summary statistics of the variables (means, standard deviations, minimum and maximum values) are to be displayed along with the correlation matrix.

cor age fimn ghqscale, means

```
. cor age fimn ghqscale, means
(obs=9613)

   Variable |       Mean   Std. Dev.          Min       Max
------------+---------------------------------------------
        age |   44.20243    18.20314           16        97
       fimn |   744.1302    743.5433     .0045041     11297
   ghqscale |   10.77125    4.914182            0        36


            |        age       fimn   ghqscale
------------+--------------------------------
        age |     1.0000
       fimn |    -0.0890     1.0000
   ghqscale |     0.0511    -0.0892     1.0000
```

If you want pairwise correlations – that is correlations between all possible cases within the data, even if they are missing on some of the variables in the variable list – then you can use the command **pwcorr**. This command displays all the pairwise correlation coefficients between the variables in the variable list or, if a variable list is not specified, between all the variables in the data set.

pwcorr age fimn ghqscale

```
. pwcorr age fimn ghqscale

            |        age       fimn   ghqscale
------------+--------------------------------
        age |     1.0000
       fimn |    -0.0969     1.0000
   ghqscale |     0.0511    -0.0892     1.0000
```

A pairwise correlation restricts the correlation to those cases which have non-missing values for the two variables under consideration. This should become clearer when you add the option **obs** below. You can see that the results here are slightly different

than the ones achieved with the **corr** command. Using the **obs**
option, we can better understand these slight discrepancies.

pwcorr age fimn ghqscale, obs

```
. pwcorr age fimn ghqscale, obs
                 |      age      fimn   ghqscale
-----------------+---------------------------------
             age |   1.0000
                 |    10264
                 |
            fimn |  -0.0969    1.0000
                 |     9912      9912
                 |
        ghqscale |   0.0511   -0.0892    1.0000
                 |     9613      9613      9613
```

You can see here how pairwise correlations allow the sample sizes
to differ. For example, we have 9613 cases in the correlation
between *age* and *ghqscale*, compared to 9912 between *age* and
fimn.

There is a variety of options that can be used with the command **pwcorr** depending upon what you want Stata to display.

- **sig** adds a line to each row of the matrix reporting the
  significance level of each correlation coefficient.
- **print(#)** specifies the significance level of correlation
  coefficients to be printed. Coefficients with larger significance
  levels are left blank. **print(.05)** would list only coefficients
  significant at the 5% level or better.
- **star(#)** specifies the significance level of coefficients to be
  starred. **star(.01)** would star all coefficients significant at
  the 1% level or better.
- **listwise** is new for version 10 and tells Stata to treat the
  missing values listwise as in the **corr** command. Therefore,
  all the **obs** values will be the same for each correlation
  reported.

Of course, these options can be combined, for example:

```
pwcorr age fimn ghqscale, obs print(.05) ///
    star(.01)
```

```
. pwcorr age fimn ghqscale, obs print(.05) ///
    star(.01)

            |      age     fimn   ghqscale
------------+------------------------------
        age |   1.0000
            |    10264
            |
       fimn |  -0.0969*   1.0000
            |    9912      9912
            |
   ghqscale |   0.0511*  -0.0892*   1.0000
            |    9613      9613      9613
```

Here you can see that the number of observations for each pair-wise correlation is printed, as well as stars. We told Stata to put stars only next to coefficients that are significant at the 0.01 level and to print correlations only if significant at the 0.05 level. Since all are starred, they are all significant at the 0.01 level. You may wonder why, especially since we told you that values below 0.30 are not considered strong enough to suggest that there is any relationship, yet values of 0.05 are considered statistically significant at the 0.01 level. An important thing to remember about significance levels with Pearson's r is that they are highly connected to sample size. Because our sample size is almost 10,000, it is more likely that associations are statistically significant. But just because a correlation is statistically significant does not mean it is substantially significant.

One way to illustrate this point is with an example. Let us run the previous command with an additional variable, the one that is the personal identification number of the respondent (*pid*).

```
pwcorr pid age fimn ghqscale, obs print(.05) ///
    star(.01)
```

```
. pwcorr pid age fimn ghqscale, obs print(.05)
    /// star(.01)
```

```
           |        pid         age        fimn    ghqscale
-----------+------------------------------------------------
       pid |    1.0000
           |     10264
           |
       age |                  1.0000
           |                  10264
           |
      fimn |   -0.0857*    -0.0969*     1.0000
           |     9912        9912        9912
           |
  ghqscale |    0.0244      0.0511*    -0.0892*     1.0000
           |     9613        9613        9613        9613
```

A researcher would never be interested in the correlation of *pid* with other variables because the values of this variable are actually nominal – they don't imply any sort of quantity. A unique number was created for everyone and its digit amount isn't important – it is just unique and allows us to follow the individual year after year. However, the output shows that it is significantly correlated with *fimn* at the 0.01 level! It is not correlated with *age* at the 0.05 level, which is why it was not printed. It was significantly correlated with *ghqscale* at the 0.05 level, which why it was printed, but not at the 0.01 level, as it was not given a star.

If you are interested in covariances instead of correlation coefficients, you can add the option **covariance** (or **cov**) after the correlation command. Covariance is a measure of how much the mean deviations of the values of two variables match. The major difference between correlation coefficients and covariance coefficients is that correlation coefficients are a scaled version of the covariance, adjusted to be between −1 and 1.

cor age fimn ghqscale, cov

```
. cor age fimn ghqscale, cov
(obs=9613)

             |         age        fimn    ghqscale
-------------+------------------------------------
         age |     331.354
        fimn |    -1204.01      552857
    ghqscale |     4.56681    -325.952     24.1492
```

Partial correlations

Before moving on, it is useful to discuss partial correlations. You may want to find out the correlation among two or more variables while controlling for the effects of a third (or more). So, for example, you might want to find out what the correlation is between age and income independently of the effects of the GHQ score.

```
pcorr age fimn ghqscale
```

```
. pcorr age fimn ghqscale
(obs=9613)

Partial correlation of age with

    Variable |      Corr.     Sig.
-------------+------------------
        fimn |    -0.0849    0.000
    ghqscale |     0.0435    0.000
```

In the results above, the partial correlations of *age* with *fimn* and *ghqscale* are given. Thus, the correlation between *age* and *fimn*, controlling for, or independent of the effects of, *ghqscale* is -0.085. Likewise, the correlation between *age* and *ghqscale*, controlling for *fimn*, is 0.044. Both are very small correlations but are statistically significant at the 0.01 level (and less). You could control for numerous interval level variables by just adding them to the variable list after the **pcorr** command.

Spearman's correlation

A non-parametric alternative to Pearson's correlation (r) is Spearman's correlation (rho). Because the four-point scales on our mental health indicators may not be 'truly' interval, it is appropriate to use a non-parametric alternative. We mean that the measure isn't 'truly' interval in the sense that the categories of response are 1 = better than usual, 2 = same as usual, 3 = less than usual, and 4 = much less than usual. We can't be certain that the distance between 1 and 2 and the distance between 3 and 4 is exactly the same. It may seem like a pedantic point, and in much real-life research ordinal variables like this (and Likert scales) are often just treated as interval level despite this violation of the assumption.

The command **spearman** followed by the variables of interest will produce the Spearman's correlation matrix.

spearman ghqa ghqb ghqc

```
. spearman ghqa ghqb ghqc
(obs=9709)

             |     ghqa      ghqb      ghqc
-------------+---------------------------
        ghqa |   1.0000
        ghqb |   0.2920   1.0000
        ghqc |   0.2500   0.1334   1.0000
```

You can also add options in a way similar to how you can in the **corr** command. For example, we can request specific statistics such as rho (the correlation coefficient), the number of observations and the *p* value associated with the estimate. You can also get Stata to only print those that are significant at 0.05 and below and to star those that are significant at the 0.01 level or less.

spearman ghqa ghqb ghqc, stats(rho obs p) ///
print(.05) star (0.01)

```
. spearman ghqa ghqb ghqc, stats(rho obs p) ///
    print(.05) star (0.01)

+--------------+
| Key          |
|--------------|
| rho          |
| Number of obs|
| Sig. level   |
+--------------+

             |     ghqa      ghqb      ghqc
-------------+---------------------------
        ghqa |   1.0000
             |   9709
             |
             |
        ghqb |   0.2920*   1.0000
             |   9709      9709
             |   0.0000
             |
        ghqc |   0.2500*   0.1334*   1.0000
             |   9709      9709      9709
             |   0.0000    0.0000
```

Pairwise correlations are also possible with the option **pw**.

```
spearman ghqa ghqb ghqc, stats(rho obs p) ///
    print(.05) star (0.01) pw
```

```
. spearman ghqa ghqb ghqc, stats(rho obs p) ///
    print(.05) star (0.01) pw
```

```
+---------------+
| Key           |
|---------------|
| rho           |
| Number of obs |
| Sig. level    |
+---------------+

             |   ghqa      ghqb      ghqc
-------------+---------------------------------
        ghqa |  1.0000
             |    9728
             |
             |
        ghqb |  0.2922*   1.0000
             |    9722      9728
             |  0.0000
             |
        ghqc |  0.2497*   0.1337*   1.0000
             |    9714      9714      9719
             |  0.0000    0.0000
```

You can see from the matrix that the request for pairwise correlations indicates that there are somewhat different numbers of respondents for each pair of correlations.

To obtain correlations by using pull-down menus, see Box 6.6.

Kendall's tau correlations

Kendall's tau and Spearman's rho are similar in some of their assumptions, but their interpretations are rather different. Spearman's rho is generally interpretable in the same way as Pearson's r (we say 'generally'; as they are computed fundamentally differently, they are obviously different statistics and not identical in their interpretation). But Kendall's tau is different. It is probably helpful to lead with an example.

> ## Box 6.6: Correlations using pull-down menus
>
> The pull-down menu equivalent of the **corr** command is:
>
> **Statistics → Summaries, tables, and tests → Summary and descriptive statistics → Correlations & covariances**
>
> The pull-down menu equivalent of the **pwcorr** command is:
>
> **Statistics → Summaries, tables, and tests → Summary and descriptive statistics → Pairwise correlations**
>
> The pull-down menu equivalent of the **pcorr** command is:
>
> **Statistics → Summaries, tables, and tests → Summary and descriptive statistics → Partial correlations**
>
> The pull-down menu equivalent of the **spearman** command is:
>
> **Statistics → Summaries, tables, and tests → Nonparametric tests of hypotheses → Spearman's rank correlation**
>
> The pull-down menu equivalent of the **ktau** command is:
>
> **Statistics → Summaries, tables, and tests → Nonparametric tests of hypotheses → Kendall's rank correlation**

We use the command **ktau**:

ktau ghqa ghqb ghqc

```
. ktau ghqa ghqb ghqc
(obs=9709)

             |     ghqa      ghqb      ghqc
-------------+---------------------------------
        ghqa |   0.3850
        ghqb |   0.1341    0.6300
        ghqc |   0.0953    0.0627    0.4179
```

Here we have a matrix of the Kendall tau correlations between all three variables. The difference with the Kendall's correlation is that while Pearson's and Spearman's correlations present results n terms of proportion of variability accounted for, Kendall's tau measures a probability: that the observed data are in the same order versus the probability that the observed data are not in same order. Its value ranges from −1 to +1. Interpretation is not straightforward, but you can request a *p* value to determine whether or not the value is statistically significant.

Other variants of Kendall's tau are available as well. The default 'tau' is technically known as Kendall's tau-a. Kendall's tau-b is often used for 2 × 2 tables but isn't limited to them.

It should be noted that **ktau** is better suited for use in small data sets as its computation time can be considerable in larger data sets.

By way of example we can show you some of the options available in the **ktau** command.

ktau ghqa ghqb ghqc, stats(taua taub p) ///
  print(.05) star (0.01)

```
ktau ghqa ghqb ghqc, stats(taua taub p) ///
   print(.05)star (0.01)
obs=9709)
```

```
------------+
  Key       |
------------|
  tau_a     |
  tau_b     |
  Sig. level|
------------+

            |    ghqa      ghqb      ghqc
------------+------------------------------
     ghqa   |  0.3850
            |  1.0000
            |
     ghqb   |  0.1341*   0.6300
            |  0.2724*   1.0000
            |  0.0000
            |
     ghqc   |  0.0953*   0.0627*   0.4179
            |  0.2376*   0.1222*   1.0000
            |  0.0000    0.0000
            |
```

We have asked Stata to report both tau-a and tau-b statistics and their significance levels, indicating that the coefficient is not printed if it is above the 0.05 level of significance and that a star is given for a significance level of were correlated at the 0.01 or less. If we were interested in the pairwise associations, we could have also added the option **pw** to the command above.

All of the correlation commands can be combined with **bysort** and **if** commands to condition the statistics reported. For example, if we want the Spearman's correlation between the three mental health items separately for men and women under 30 years old:

bysort sex: spearman ghqa ghqb ghqc if age<30

```
. bysort sex: spearman ghqa ghqb ghqc if age<30

------------------------------------------------------------
-> sex = male
(obs=1211)

             |     ghqa     ghqb     ghqc
-------------+------------------------------
        ghqa |   1.0000
        ghqb |   0.2470   1.0000
        ghqc |   0.2070   0.0786   1.0000


------------------------------------------------------------
-> sex = female
(obs=1281)

             |     ghqa     ghqb     ghqc
-------------+------------------------------
        ghqa |   1.0000
        ghqb |   0.2740   1.0000
        ghqc |   0.1954   0.0989   1.0000
```

TWO-VARIABLE GRAPHS

As we have done previously, we start looking at graphs by using the pull-down menus. First, we produce a scatterplot of monthly income against age by selecting:

Graphics → Twoway graph

This brings up the **twoway - Twoway graphs** dialogue box. This is for simple scatterplots and for more complicated overlaid two-way graphs (see Box 6.7). This dialogue box is completely new for version 10, so if you're using version 9 you either use the **Easy graphs** pull-down menu choices or the more detailed **Scatterplot** option.

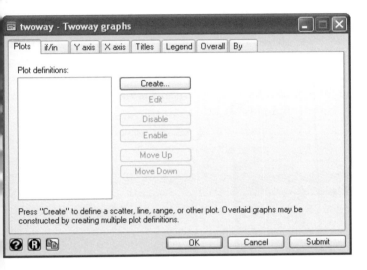

To make a scatterplot, or any other two variable graph, you first click the **Create** button and this brings up a new dialogue box named **Plot 1** in which you specify which variables to use and what type of graph. In this example we choose the type of graph – **Scatter** with **Basic plots** selected – and then either scroll down to or type in the X and Y variables – in this case *age* and *fimn*, respectively.

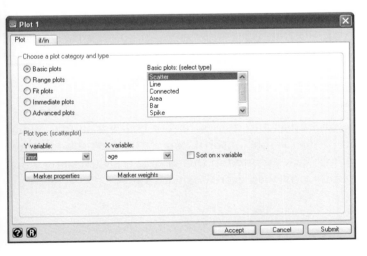

When you have finished creating the graph, click on the **Accept** button and the **Plot 1** dialogue box will close and return you to the **twoway – Twoway graphs** dialogue box. You can see that this now has Plot 1 in the **Plot definitions** box and you are able to change the plot by clicking on the **Edit** button which will bring up the **Plot 1** dialogue box again. The other tabs are fairly self-explanatory if you have read Chapter 5.

Remember that although many of the functions in the tabs can now be done in the Graph Editor once the basic graph is created, the Graph Editor does not produce a command. So we suggest doing as much as possible in the commands or pull-down menus, leaving only minor changes/additions to the Graph Editor.

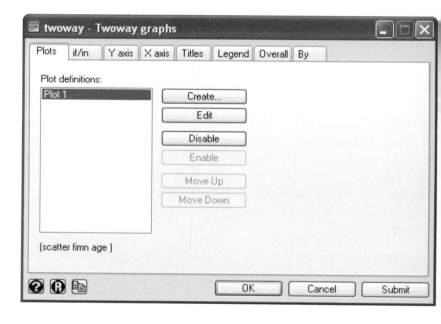

Click on the **OK** button and the scatterplot below is shown, which you can edit in the Graph Editor if you wish. Even though there are thousands of cases plotted in this graph, it clearly shows that income generally rises then decreases with age.

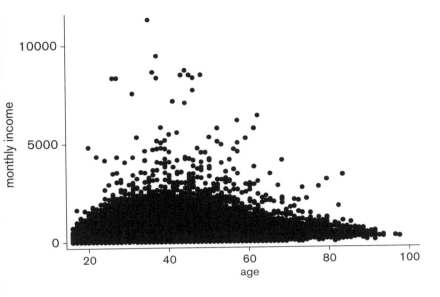

Box 6.7: Overlaid two variable graphs

In this demonstration we wish to plot income (*fimn*) against mental health (*ghqscale*) separately for men and women but overlaid on the same axes in order to compare the distributions. We restrict the graphing to those who are aged 40 so that there will be a small number of cases plotted and so that you can see the difference more clearly. We also restrict the cases to those earning less than £3000 per month, which removes the outliers so the income scale is more manageable.

Follow the same pull-down menu path as for simple scatterplots:

Graphics → Twoway graph

This time we need to create two new plots in the Plot definitions box. First create a plot (or edit Plot 1 if one is still listed there from previous work) that specifies a scatterplot with *fimn* on the X axis and *ghqscale* on the Y axis. For Plot 1 use the **if/in** tab to restrict this plot to men (sex==1), aged 40 (age==40), with income less than £3000 (fimn<3000). Below is the dialogue box for Plot 2 which has the same specifications as Plot 1 except that sex==2, so this plot is restricted to women.

▶

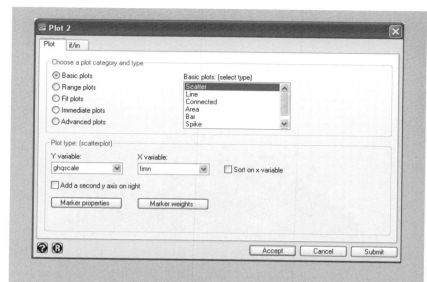

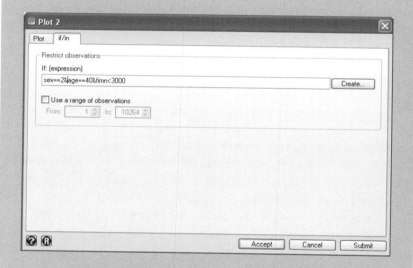

If you now produce the scatterplot you will see that the legend doesn't make any sense when it should tell you which symbols are for men and which are for women. Either you can change this in the **Legend** tab as shown below (click on the **?** button for help on what to type in the **Override default keys** box) or in the **Chart Editor**; you know that men are the first plot and therefore the first in the legend from left to right or top to bottom (depending how your legend is formatted).

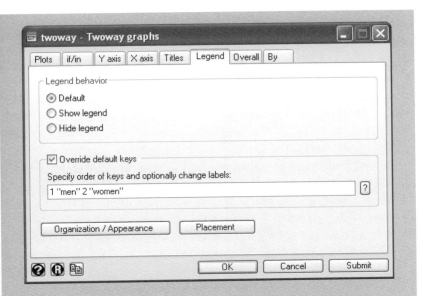

This produces an overlaid scatterplot in which the circles are men and diamonds are women. We have changed the scheme to a monochrome one for better printing in black and white. To change the style of the graph use the pull-down menu **Edit → Apply new scheme** when the chart first appears, before opening the **Chart Editor**. Try out some of the different schemes available to see which ones are most suitable for your uses.

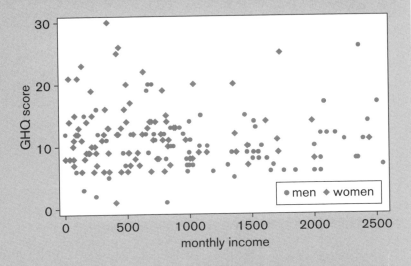

You may have noticed that Stata 'echoes' the commands in the Results window when you use the pull-down menus to ▶

▶ create graphs. But it is worth noting that any changes done through the Graph Editor are not echoed in the Results window. So if you have found a graph that you want to replicate simply copy the command from the Results window and paste it into a do file.

An extension to these graphs is to add a third variable on a right-hand Y axis. In this example we plot *age* on the X axis and then *ghqscale* on the left Y axis and *fimn* on the right Y axis. We restrict the sample to self-employed women. If you look back to the first screen capture in this box, you will notice that in Plot 2 there is an option to **Add a second y axis on right**. For Plot 1 we use *ghqscale* on the Y axis and for Plot 2 we use *fimn* on the Y axis. In both plots we specify `sex==2&jbstat==1` in the if/in tab. Don't forget to remove or edit the legend labels if you are following on from the previous example.

This produces the scatterplot below, where we have changed the output to monochrome for better printing in black and white. As you can imagine with the capabilities of Stata, these graphs can be very complex. Enjoy exploring the possibilities!

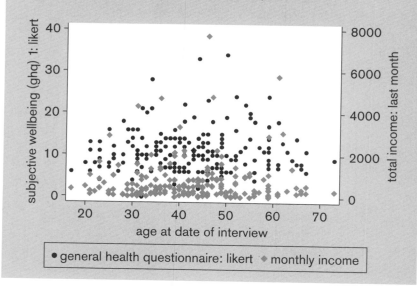

You may notice in the main **Graphics** pull-down menu and there is something called **Scatterplot matrix**.

Graphics → **Scatterplot matrix**

If the three interval level variables (*age*, *fimn*, *ghqscale*) in the example data are entered into the box, Stata produces a matrix of scatterplots of each pair of variables. It's a quick way to inspect the association between a number of variables.

The next type of two-variable graph we introduce here is the bar chart. Stata differentiates between bar charts and histograms (see Chapter 5 for histograms). Bar charts produce a summary of one variable by categories of another. In our example we graph mean scores of the *ghqscale* variable by categories of the health status variable (*hlstat*).

Graphics → Bar chart

In the **Main** tab we put *ghqscale* in the **Variables** box and then choose the statistic we want to summarize that variable; the default for the first row is the mean. Note here that you can put more than one variable in the **Variables** box, but make sure the scales of those variables are comparable.

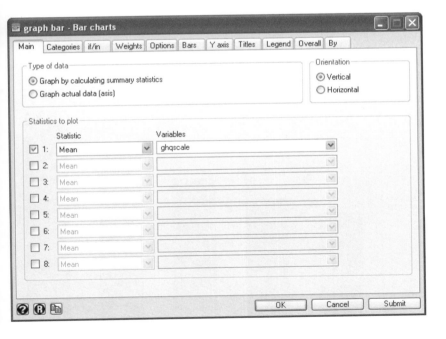

The categorical variable that will form the X axis is entered in Group 1 box of the **Categories** tab, in this example *hlstat*.

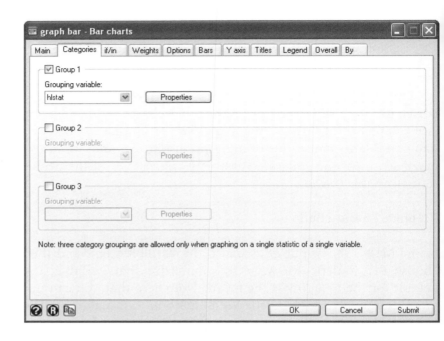

This produces the following bar chart which shows quite clearly an increasing mean of GHQ score as self-reported health gets worse.

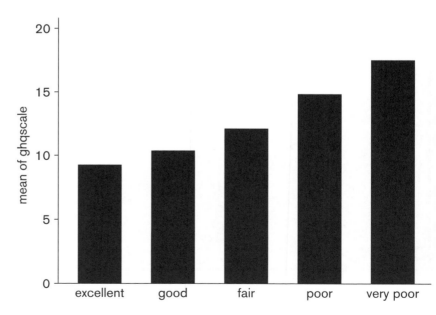

In the **Categories** tab you can see that there is space for other 'grouping' variables. Depending on how you enter the variables in the Group 1 and Group 2 boxes, different chart formats will result, as can be seen the two charts below. In the top chart Group 1 is *hlstat* and Group 2 is *sex*. In the bottom chart Group 1 is *sex* and Group 2 is *hlstat*.

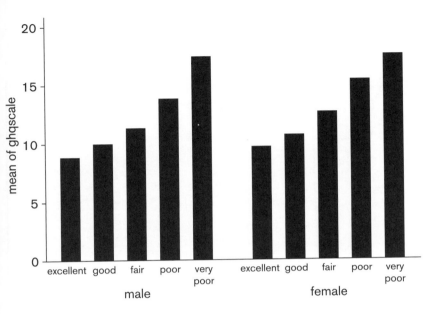

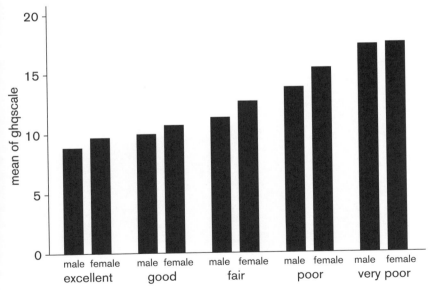

The third type of two-variable graph we cover in this chapter is grouped box plots. If you revise the creation of box plots in Chapter 5 you will remember that there is a **Categories** tab in the **graph box – Box plots** dialogue box that opens when selecting:

Graphics → Box plot

So after putting the variable you wish to summarize in the box plots in the **Main** tab, put the categorical variable in the **Categories** tab. You can have up to three grouping variables, but in this example we have used two: *hlstat* and *sex*. These grouping variables operate in the same way as in bar charts above.

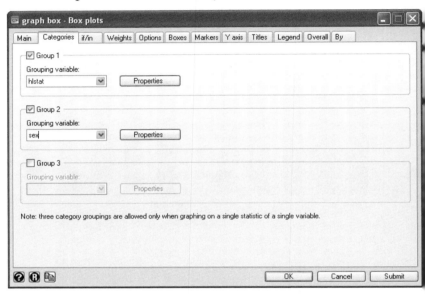

The resulting box plot now plots GHQ score for each category of health status and for both men and women separately.

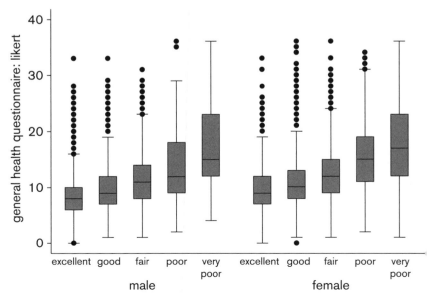

DEMONSTRATION EXERCISE

In Chapter 3 we manipulated the individual level variables and saved a new data set called demodata1.dta. In Chapter 4 we merged a household level variable indicating the region of the country onto the individual level data and saved the data with a new name demodata2.dta. In Chapter 5 we examined the variables we are using for their distribution, measures of central tendency and, for interval variables, their normality.

At this stage of this demonstration we start exploring the associations between our outcome variable (*ghqscale*) and the factors believed to affect mental health. As the *ghqscale* variable is interval level, we can look for differences in mean scores across categories in the other variables: *female, agecat, marst2, empstat, numchd* and *region2*. This can be done with a single command using **tab1** and the **su** option:

```
tab1 female agecat marst2 empstat numchd ///
    region2, su(ghq)
```

Note that we have used *ghq* instead of the full name of the variable *ghqscale*. Stata allows you to shorten variable names provided that the shortening only identifies one variable. In other words, if we had two variables that started with the letters *ghq* then Stata would return an error.

```
. tab1 female agecat marst2 empstat numchd ///
    region2, su(ghq)

-> tabulation of female
    female |        Summary of ghq 0-36
 indicator |       Mean      Std. Dev.       Freq.
-----------+-------------------------------------
      male |   10.197257      4.7327355        3645
    female |   11.315802      5.0705736        4069
-----------+-------------------------------------
     Total |    10.78727      4.9451537        7714

-> tabulation of agecat
       age |        Summary of ghq 0-36
categories |       Mean      Std. Dev.       Freq.
-----------+-------------------------------------
 18-32 yea |   10.563872      4.8776024        2779
 33-50 yea |    11.03622      4.9563576        3175
 51-65 yea |   10.690909      5.0129936        1760
-----------+-------------------------------------
     Total |    10.78727      4.9451537        7714
```

```
-> tabulation of marst2

   marital |
  status 4 |           Summary of ghq 0-36
categories |         Mean     Std. Dev.       Freq.
-----------+-------------------------------------
    single |    10.345222      5.010017        1486
   married |    10.677812     4.7087427        5503
   sep/div |    12.638182     6.2309817         550
   widowed |    12.165714      5.603875         175
-----------+-------------------------------------
     Total |     10.78727     4.9451537        7714

-> tabulation of empstat

employment |           Summary of ghq 0-36
    status |         Mean     Std. Dev.       Freq.
-----------+-------------------------------------
  employed |    10.254293     4.4085201        5474
unemploye  |    12.934959      6.091281         492
  longterm |    15.365957     6.8533252         235
  studying |    10.375566     5.0631593         221
family ca  |    12.119183     5.6297188         881
   retired |    10.002597     4.5492094         385
-----------+-------------------------------------
     Total |    10.786681     4.9406805        7688

-> tabulation of numchd

children 3 |           Summary of ghq 0-36
categories |         Mean     Std. Dev.       Freq.
-----------+-------------------------------------
      none |    10.555601      4.926495        4874
one or tw  |    11.174229     4.9786735        2336
  three or |    11.234127     4.8349237         504
-----------+-------------------------------------
     Total |     10.78727     4.9451537        7714

-> tabulation of region2

 regions 7 |           Summary of ghq 0-36
categories |         Mean     Std. Dev.       Freq.
-----------+-------------------------------------
    London |    10.911873     5.1982339         817
     South |    10.615874      4.649652        2356
  Midlands |    10.797145     5.0592898        1331
 Northwest |    10.753086     4.8014493         810
 North and |    10.825739     5.0068762        1251
     Wales |    11.605528     5.6338908         398
  Scotland |    10.711052     4.9890945         751
-----------+-------------------------------------
     Total |     10.78727     4.9451537        7714
```

If we didn't want to see the standard deviation and frequencies then we could add the **means** option so that Stata only produces the mean *ghqscale* value for each category:

tab1 female agecat marst2 empstat numchd ///
    region2,su(ghq) means

```
.  tab1 female agecat marst2 empstat numchd ///
      region2,su(ghq) means

-> tabulation of female

           | Summary of
    female |  ghq 0-36
 indicator |      Mean
-----------+------------
      male |   10.197257
    female |   11.315802
-----------+------------
     Total |   10.78727

-> tabulation of agecat

           | Summary of
       age |  ghq 0-36
categories |      Mean
-----------+------------
18-32 yea  |   10.563872
33-50 yea  |   11.03622
51-65 yea  |   10.690909
-----------+------------
     Total |   10.78727
```

Etc.

However, we would suggest that it is useful to see the number of cases in each category so you can see if any variations in mean values are based on categories with a small number of cases.

As you can see from the first output there are some potential differences in mean GHQ scores between males and females, across categories of marital status, employment status, and number of children in the household. The variations across age categories look small, as do the variations across regions. We will formally test these differences in the next chapter.

In addition to using age categories, we have the interval level measure of age in the data set. In this case we can correlate the two interval level variables: *ghqscale* and *age*.

```
pwcorr ghq age, sig
```

. pwcorr ghqscale age, sig

```
             |  ghqscale       age
-------------+--------------------
   ghqscale  |    1.0000
             |
             |
        age  |    0.0123    1.0000
             |    0.2800
             |
```

We have used the **pwcorr** command so that we can use the **sig** option which will display the p value in the output. Pearson's r is 0.012 and the p value is 0.28, which indicates that there is a very small and statistically non-significant linear association between these two variables. As Pearson's r relates to a linear association there is the possibility that this low correlation disguises a non-linear association. The means tables indicated that the mean GHQ score for the middle age group was higher than the other two. To further investigate if a non-linear association exists we first graph the two variables.

Graphics → Twoway graph

We put *age* as the X variable and *ghqscale* as the Y variable and Stata produces this scatterplot. As there are over 7000 cases it is difficult to distinguish any pattern.

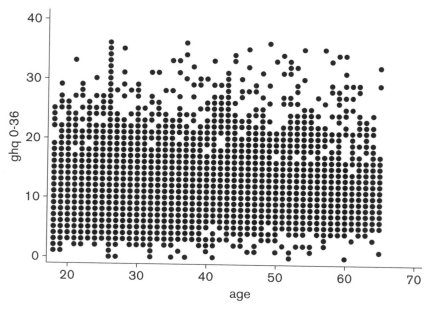

An alternative approach is to graph the mean GHQ values for each age to see the pattern. This can be done in a number of ways but in this exercise we use the bar chart.

Graphics → Bar charts

This brings up the bar chart dialogue box where the default statistic is the mean which we want to use. In the **Variables** tab we either type or scroll down and select the *ghqscale* variable, and in the **Categories** tab we choose *age* as the Group 1 variable. This produces:

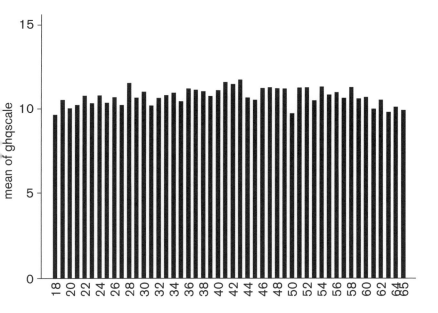

This bar chart is not exactly neat, but it serves the purpose of letting us examine the mean GHQ score at each age. It appears to generally rise as age increases then fall slightly. We test whether a non-linear association captures this information better than a linear one in Chapter 8.

Returning to the point of having two 'Grouping' variables, we can use that option to inspect the age distribution of mean GHQ scores for both men and women. This time we use the age categories rather than age in years as the Group 1 variable and *female* as the Group 2 variable. We also orientate the labels of the age categories so that they don't run into each other and thus make the graph more readable.

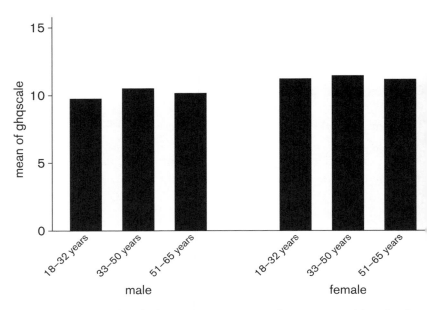

Next we use the dichotomous GHQ indicator variable (*d_ghq*) in crosstabs with the nominal or ordinal variables and test whether there is a statistical association. In this example we start off by using the most applicable test statistic – chi-squared – by using a series of **tab** commands. We use the **nofreq** option as we just wish to see the statistics before we go any further in our investigation.

```
ta d_ghq female, chi2 nofreq
ta d_ghq agecat, chi2 nofreq
ta d_ghq marst2, chi2 nofreq
ta d_ghq empstat, chi2 nofreq
ta d_ghq numchd, chi2 nofreq
ta d_ghq region2, chi2 nofreq
```

```
. ta d_ghq female, chi2 nofreq
        Pearson chi2(1) = 25.7939  Pr = 0.000

. ta d_ghq agecat, chi2 nofreq
        Pearson chi2(2) = 6.4265   Pr = 0.040

. ta d_ghq marst2, chi2 nofreq
        Pearson chi2(3) = 53.3636  Pr = 0.000

. ta d_ghq empstat, chi2 nofreq
        Pearson chi2(5) = 284.0623 Pr = 0.000
```

```
. ta d_ghq numchd, chi2 nofreq
         Pearson chi2(2) = 10.8155   Pr = 0.004

. ta d_ghq region2, chi2 nofreq
         Pearson chi2(6) = 17.3147   Pr = 0.008
```

As you can see from this output, there are significant associations ($p < 0.05$) between the independent variables and the dichotomous GHQ variable. The chi-squared test only tells you that there are different distributions across the categories, but it doesn't tell us where these variations are. We test for these in the next chapter.

At this stage we want to examine some of these variations in more detail to help inform our future analyses. In this demonstration we examine the association between age categories and the dichotomous GHQ indicator. First we produce a full crosstabulation with percentages:

ta agecat d_ghq, row chi2

```
. ta agecat d_ghq, row chi2

+----------------+
| Key            |
|----------------|
| frequency      |
| row percentage |
+----------------+

        age |        d_ghq
 categories |       0          1 |    Total
------------+--------------------+---------
18-32 years |    2,233        546 |    2,779
            |    80.35      19.65 |   100.00
------------+--------------------+---------
33-50 years |    2,572        603 |    3,175
            |    81.01      18.99 |   100.00
------------+--------------------+---------
51-65 years |    1,466        294 |    1,760
            |    83.30      16.70 |   100.00
------------+--------------------+---------
      Total |    6,271      1,443 |    7,714
            |    81.29      18.71 |   100.00

        Pearson chi2(2) = 6.4265   Pr = 0.040
```

This shows that the percentage of those over the GHQ threshold decreases with age – from 19.6% in the youngest category to 16.7% in the oldest category. If we look back to the bar chart of mean *ghqscale* values by age and gender above, as well as take into account the significant differences between males and females in the dichotomous GHQ indicator, it might be useful to break out this table by gender using the **bysort** command:

bysort female:ta agecat d_ghq, row chi2

```
. bysort female:ta agecat d_ghq, row chi2

------------------------------------------------------------------
-> female = male

+----------------+
| Key            |
|----------------|
| frequency      |
| row percentage |
+----------------+


          age |        d_ghq
   categories |       0         1 |     Total
--------------+------------------+----------
  18-32 years |   1,104       203 |     1,307
              |   84.47     15.53 |    100.00
--------------+------------------+----------
  33-50 years |   1,235       263 |     1,498
              |   82.44     17.56 |    100.00
--------------+------------------+----------
  51-65 years |     711       129 |       840
              |   84.64     15.36 |    100.00
--------------+------------------+----------
        Total |   3,050       595 |     3,645
              |   83.68     16.32 |    100.00

      Pearson chi2(2) = 2.8421   Pr = 0.241
```

```
-----------------------------------------------------

-> female = female

+-----------------+
| Key             |
|-----------------|
| frequency       |
| row percentage  |
+-----------------+

       age  |         d_ghq
  categories |        0          1 |     Total
-----------+-------------------+---------
18-32 years |    1,129        343 |     1,472
            |    76.70      23.30 |    100.00
-----------+-------------------+---------
33-50 years |    1,337        340 |     1,677
            |    79.73      20.27 |    100.00
-----------+-------------------+---------
51-65 years |      755        165 |       920
            |    82.07      17.93 |    100.00
-----------+-------------------+---------
      Total |    3,221        848 |     4,069
            |    79.16      20.84 |    100.00

     Pearson chi2(2) = 10.4390   Pr = 0.005
```

This output shows that the original association was largely driven by the differences in age categories and GHQ indicator for females. The chi-squared test shows that for males there is no significant association ($p = 0.241$), whereas for females there is significant association ($p = 0.005$). An inspection of the percentages reported in the crosstabulations confirms this with only small differences for males, while females show considerably more reduction in the percentage over the GHQ threshold – from 23.3% in the youngest age category to 17.9% in the oldest age category.

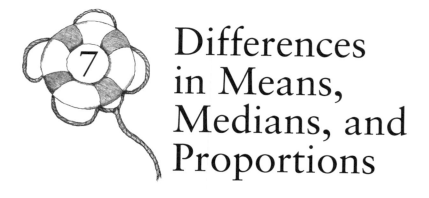

Differences in Means, Medians, and Proportions

In the previous chapter, we explored different types of tables and correlations: statistical analyses that tell us about associations between variables. In this chapter, we focus on tests that tell us something slightly different: whether there are groups that have different means, medians, ranks, or proportions.

T-TESTS

This family of tests has a common feature in that they compare the means of variables between two groups. In order to compare the means of a variable between two groups, two very specific conditions must be met:

- the variable whose mean difference you're interested in must be measured at the interval level, and
- there cannot be more that two groups on which you are comparing the mean value – the grouping variable must be *dichotomous*.

The most common type of *t*-test is usually just called a '*t*-test', but is also known as the independent samples *t*-test, independent two-samples *t*-test, the Student's *t*-test, and Student's independent samples *t*-test. They all mean the same thing.

Independent two-samples *t*-test
The name of the independent two-samples *t*-test can be a bit confusing for the statistical novice. Some might think that 'two samples' means you need to be using different data sets. This

is not the case. 'Two samples' just means that there are two non-overlapping groups in your data – such as men and women, or ethnic minorities and non-minorities. It is typical that before you begin any major analysis you might want to see if there are any mean differences in your data that might be interesting to pursue with more sophisticated techniques (such as multivariate analysis, covered in the next chapter).

Suppose we want to compare the average age of men and women in our data. We would perform a *t*-test for the differences between means in age between men and women. This is done by using the command **ttest**. After the command **ttest** you put the interval variable. The **by** option specifies the groups we want to compare. Note that is it important to include the parentheses around the dichotomous variable.

ttest age, by(sex)

```
. ttest age, by(sex)

Two-sample t test with equal variances
-------------------------------------------------------------------------
  Group |     Obs      Mean  Std. Err.  Std. Dev.  [95% Conf. Interval]
--------+----------------------------------------------------------------
   male |    4833  43.26381  .2585778   17.97627   42.75688   43.77074
 female |    5431  45.44043  .2553488   18.81801   44.93985   45.94102
--------+----------------------------------------------------------------
combined|   10264  44.41553  .1821865   18.45757   44.05841   44.77265
--------+----------------------------------------------------------------
   diff |           -2.176623  .3643778            -2.890875  -1.462372
-------------------------------------------------------------------------
    diff = mean(male) - mean(female)                    t =  -5.9735
Ho: diff = 0                             degrees of freedom =    10262

    Ha: diff < 0              Ha: diff != 0                Ha: diff > 0
Pr(T < t) = 0.0000     Pr(|T| > |t|) = 0.0000       Pr(T > t) = 1.0000
```

The output gives you a lot of information. First of all, you can see that there are 4833 males and 5431 females in the sample. The mean age of males was 43.26 years, while it was 45.44 years for females. The next columns report the standard error of the mean, the standard deviation, and the 95% confidence intervals of the mean.

Underneath, you see a combined mean of 44.42, which is the average age of all males and females, with the associated standard error, standard deviation and confidence interval. The next row tells you that the difference between the average ages of males and females was just over two years (2.18), and this figure also has a standard error and confidence interval.

But are the means significantly different from one another? This is where the report at the bottom of the table comes into play. You will see that Stata reports that we were testing diff=mean(male) – mean(female) and that the associated *t* statistic is −5.97. There is also a line that says the hypothesis

Box 7.1: Critical values

If you go to a statistics book and look at a table of critical values of *t* for a two-tailed test at the .95 level of significance with *n* − 2 degrees of freedom (in this case 10,262, but in the table you will likely find 120 or 'infinity'), you will see a critical value of ±1.96. If you look for the critical value of corresponding to a one-tailed test at the .95 level of significance, you will see a critical value of ±1.645. The *t* calculated in our estimation is −5.9735. This value is below −1.96 on the *t* distribution as well as much below −1.645 (with a two-tailed test, you can look at either the positive or negative value, i.e. both sides of the 'the tail'). Therefore if we were testing the hypothesis that Ha != 0 or that Ha: diff < 0, we would be able to reject the null. If we had a one-tailed test and our hypothesis was that Ha: diff > 0, we would have to fail to reject the null because our critical value of *t* would be 1.645 and our *t* statistic is −5.97. For one-tailed tests we look at one side of the *t* distribution only. The figures below illustrate the hypotheses and critical values associated with the alternative hypotheses.

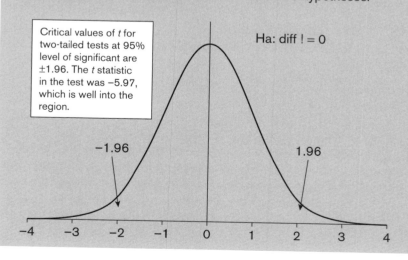

Critical values of *t* for two-tailed tests at 95% level of significant are ±1.96. The *t* statistic in the test was −5.97, which is well into the region.

Ha: diff ! = 0

−1.96

1.96

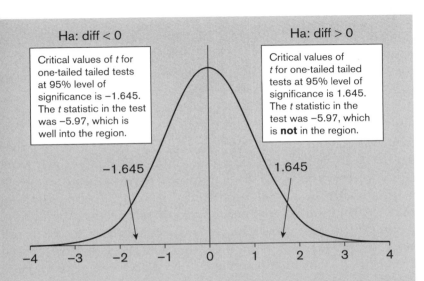

Ha: diff < 0

Critical values of *t* for one-tailed tailed tests at 95% level of significance is −1.645. The *t* statistic in the test was −5.97, which is well into the region.

Ha: diff > 0

Critical values of *t* for one-tailed tailed tests at 95% level of significance is 1.645. The *t* statistic in the test was −5.97, which is **not** in the region.

−1.645

1.645

It should be noted that, in practice, most social scientists report two-tailed tests, although scientifically it is perfectly acceptable to examine tests from a one-tailed perspective if theory or previous research gives you some reasons to test hypotheses directionally. You can also see that when tests are one-tailed, the critical value of *t* is a smaller value, thus making it 'easier' for a test statistic to achieve statistical significance. In the previous example, the findings were significant using a one- or two-tailed test. Imagine if the test statistic had been −1.75. It would have been significant with the one-tailed test where we need a smaller value than −1.645 to be statistically significant, but not the two-tailed test, where the test statistic would fail to be smaller than −1.96.

being tested is Ho: diff = 0. That is, the null hypothesis is that the difference between the two means is zero (in other words, there is no difference). You will probably recall that the null hypothesis is something that we are essentially trying to disprove or find evidence against.

There are three alternative hypotheses listed: Ha: diff < 0, Ha: diff != 0, and Ha: diff > 0. While your null hypothesis is that there is no difference between the means, there are three possible alternatives to this: that the difference between the two will be less than zero, that the difference is greater than zero, or that the difference in means is just somehow different from zero. So if you had some reason to hypothesize that men would be younger than women, then the alternative hypothesis you would test would be Ha: `diff < 0`. If you thought that men would be older than the women in the sample, then the hypothesis you would be testing is Ha: `diff > 0`. However, if you are simply testing there will be some kind of difference in ages, your hypothesis is Ha: `diff != 0` (remember that != means not equal to).

The major difference here is that the hypotheses Ha: `diff < 0` and Ha: `diff > 0` are one-tailed or directional hypotheses. This means that you are looking for a specific result that is either greater than or less than zero and you have a reason (be it from theory or previous research) that the difference in means will be in a *specific* direction. With a one-tailed test, the critical region on the *t*-distribution is on one side, or one 'tail' of the distribution. A two-tailed test means that you suspect a difference exists, but you are not sure what the direction will be. Thus, the critical regions that your hypothesis tests are in both tail areas of the *t* distribution.

One of the assumptions of a *t*-test is that the groups have equal variances. You can test for this by using a number of commands that are detailed in the section on one-way ANOVA. If your groups do not have equal variances you need to specify the option **unequal** in your **ttest** command. See Box 7.2 for *t*-tests using pull-down menus.

If you wish to use the **ttest** command to test for differences between two categories of a categorical variable with more than two categories then you need to condition the command with an **if** statement. For example, if you wanted to test for differences in mean ages for those who are cohabiting (*mastat*=2) and those widowed (*mastat*=3) then you would use:

ttest age if mastat==2 | mastat==3,by(mastat)

```
. ttest age if mastat==2 | mastat==3,by(mastat)
Two-sample t test with equal variances
-------------------------------------------------------------------------------
  Group |    Obs      Mean   Std. Err.  Std. Dev.  [95% Conf. Interval]
--------+----------------------------------------------------------------------
living a |    674  32.37834  .4674598   12.13596    31.46048   33.29619
 widowed |    866  72.18245  .3766843   11.08502    71.44313   72.92177
--------+----------------------------------------------------------------------
combined |   1540  54.76169  .5831274   22.88357    53.61788   55.9055
--------+----------------------------------------------------------------------
    diff |         -39.80411  .5936135              -40.96849  -38.63973
-------------------------------------------------------------------------------
    diff = mean(living a) - mean(widowed)                    t = -67.0539
Ho: diff = 0                                degrees of freedom =    1538

   Ha: diff < 0              Ha: diff != 0                Ha: diff > 0
Pr(T < t) = 0.0000    Pr(|T| > |t|) = 0.0000       Pr(T > t) = 1.0000
```

Box 7.2: Independent two-sample *t*-tests using pull-down menus

Through the pull-down menus, you can also get to the same results by going to:

Statistics → Summaries, tables and tests → Classical tests of hypotheses → Two-group mean-comparison test

Then you fill in the dialogue box like this:

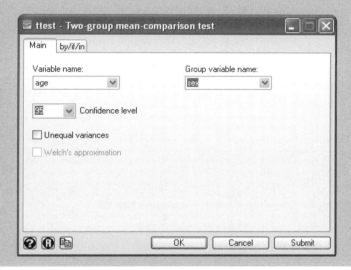

One sample *t*-test

You may also want to perform a one sample *t*-test where you are testing if the mean of a variable is statistically different from some specific value that is specified a priori (see Box 7.3 for the pull-down menu for this test). You may have a value in mind from previous research or theory. Let us suppose that we have a belief that the average number of hours worked (*jbhrs*) among sample members is 35 hours per week.

```
ttest jbhrs=35
```

```
. ttest jbhrs=35

One-sample t test
-----------------------------------------------------------------------
Variable |   Obs       Mean   Std. Err.   Std. Dev.   [95% Conf. Interval]
---------+-------------------------------------------------------------
   jbhrs |   5260   33.64449    .173371    12.57388    33.30461   33.98437
-----------------------------------------------------------------------
    mean = mean(jbhrs)                                    t =  -7.8180
Ho: mean = 35                               degrees of freedom =    5259

  Ha: mean < 35                 Ha: mean != 35                 Ha: mean > 35
Pr(T < t) = 0.0000        Pr(|T| > |t|) = 0.0000        Pr(T > t) = 1.0000
```

The results indicate that the sample mean is 33.64, which is significantly less than (and different from) 35, as indicated by the results for the alternative hypotheses Ha: mean < 35 and Ha: mean != 35.

Box 7.3: One sample *t*-test using pull-down menus

Through the pull-down menus, you can also get to the same results by going to:

Statistics → Summaries, tables and tests → Classical tests of hypotheses → One-sample mean-comparison test

Then fill in this dialogue box:

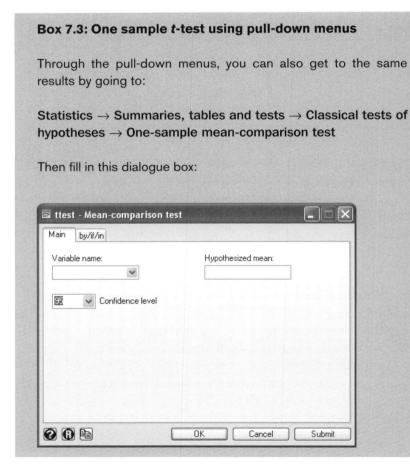

Similarly to the written commands, we can click on the **by/if/in** tab in the dialogue box and select and fill in the option to **Repeat command by groups**.

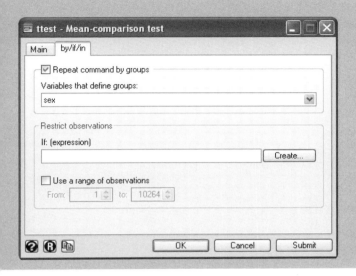

You could also test this mean difference by sex (or any other categorical variable). For example, you could see if hours worked were statistically different from 35 for both sexes using the **bysort** command.

bysort sex: ttest jbhrs=35

Mann–Whitney *U*-test

The Mann–Whitney *U*-test is the nonparametric version of the independent samples *t*-test. You would use the *U*-test to examine *rank* differences across some characteristic for two groups. This test is particularly appropriate if your variable of interest is ordinal rather than interval. Recall that the level of measurement required for the independent samples *t*-test is interval. The command for the Mann–Whitney *U*-test is **ranksum** (see Box 7.4 for pull-down menu instructions). This test is also known as the Mann–Whitney two-sample test.

Let's pick an ordinal variable, such as self-reported health status (*hlstat*), which has five response categories: excellent, good, fair, poor, and very poor. We can see if the rank ordering differs by sex. We put the grouping variable, in this case *sex*, in parentheses after the **by** option in a similar way to the **ttest** command.

ranksum hlstat, by(sex)

```
. ranksum hlstat, by(sex)

Two-sample Wilcoxon rank-sum (Mann-Whitney)
test
```

sex	obs	rank sum	expected
male	4832	23683134	24780912
female	5424	28914762	27816984
combined	10256	52597896	52597896

```
unadjusted variance        2.240e+10
adjustment for ties       -2.699e+09
                           --------
adjusted variance          1.970e+10

Ho: hlstat(sex==male) = hlstat(sex==female)

        z =  -7.821
Prob > |z| =   0.0000
```

Box 7.4: Mann–Whitney *U*-test using pull-down menus

In the pull-down menus go to:

Statistics → Summaries, tables and tests → Nonparametric
tests of hypotheses → Wilcoxon ranksum test

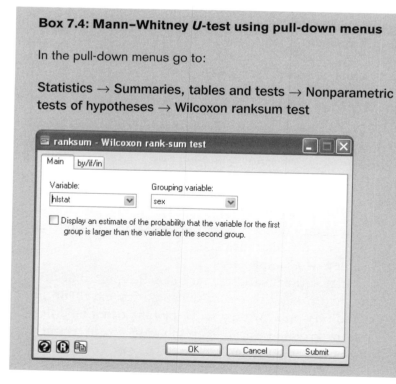

You will notice that at the top of the output, it states that this is a two-sample Wilcoxon rank-sum test, but the results note that it is also known as Mann–Whitney. Our results first tell us the number of results for males and females, and then their 'rank sum' compared to their 'expected' sum. These are the figures that are computed when the data points for males' and females' health status scores are converted to ranks – the expected column is the figure that would be expected if there was no relationship between the variable of interest (*hlstat*) and the group variable (*sex*).

There are three variance statistics reported: unadjusted, adjusted for ties, and the overall adjusted variance. However, more importantly, the next rows tell us the null hypothesis that was tested and the statistical significance of our test statistic.

We were testing the null hypothesis that the overall rank of men's health status was the same as for females. The associated *z* statistic for this was –7.821, for which the associated *p* value was 0.00, which is statistically significant (i.e. it is much smaller than the typical 0.05 cut-off figure). As the test statistic is negative, we know that females' self-reported health was significantly *worse* than that of males. Higher scores on the self-reported health score were associated with 'poor' and 'very poor' health, and we know that the ranks of females subtracted from ranks of males resulted in a negative score, as evidenced by the *z* statistic.

Non-parametric equality-of-medians test

A similar test to the Mann–Whitney *U*-test is the non-parametric equality-of-medians test, which is the command **median** (see Box 7.5 for pull-down menu instructions). We can perform the same estimation as above using this command instead.

median hlstat, by(sex)

```
. median hlstat, by(sex)
Median test

Greater than |         sex
  the median |    male    female |    Total
-------------+------------------+---------
          no |   3,685     3,858 |    7,543
         yes |   1,147     1,566 |    2,713
-------------+------------------+---------
       Total |   4,832     5,424 |   10,256

     Pearson chi2(1) =  34.6226   Pr = 0.000
  Continuity corrected:
     Pearson chi2(1) =  34.3592   Pr = 0.000
```

You can see from the results that the output is organized differently such that we are given information about number of cases greater than the median by *sex*. Pearson's chi-squared statistics are reported, with a 'continuity correction' (correction for small samples). In any case, we can see that we have statistically significant results as the *p* value (here reported as **Pr**) is 0.000. It is rather hard to tell from the results table what the differences are exactly, however.

It should be noted that with the **median** command the number of categories that we may examine our ordinal variable by is not limited to two, as in the **ranksum** command. Thus, this command is also a non-parametric alternative to the one-way analysis of variance, which we discuss later in this chapter.

Box 7.5: Non-parametric equality-of-medians test using pull-down menus

Through the pull-down menus, we can also get to the same results by going to:

Statistics → Summaries, tables and tests → Nonparametric tests of hypotheses → K-sample equality-of-medians test

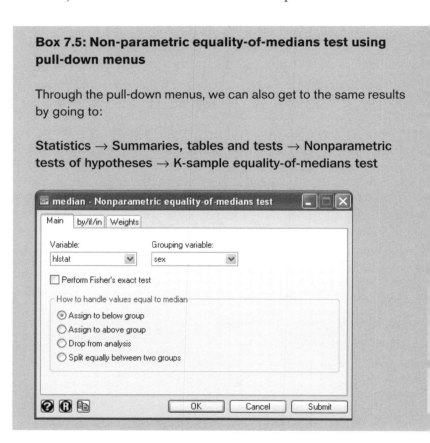

One- and two-sample tests of proportions

In Chapter 3 we discussed dummy variables at length. Dummy variables themselves are dichotomous indicators but also represent proportions when summed across categories. Let's tabulate whether or not someone attended university (where yes = 1 and no = 0) by their sex.

```
. ta university sex, col

+-------------------+
| Key               |
|-------------------|
|      frequency    |
| column percentage |
+-------------------+

           |         sex
university |    male   female |    Total
-----------+------------------+---------
         0 |   4,425    5,119 |    9,544
           |   91.56    94.26 |    92.99
-----------+------------------+---------
         1 |     408      312 |      720
           |    8.44     5.74 |     7.01
-----------+------------------+---------
     Total |   4,833    5,431 |   10,264
           |  100.00   100.00 |   100.00
```

You can see that 8.44% of all males went to university compared to 5.74% of females. This difference looks sizeable, but is it statistically significant? This is where a test of proportions is used (see Box 7.6 for the pull-down menu equivalent).

prtest university, by(sex)

```
. prtest university, by(sex)

Two-sample test of proportion male:         Number of obs = 4833
                                    female: Number of obs = 5431

------------------------------------------------------------------
Variable |    Mean   Std. Err.    z    P>|z|   [95% Conf. Interval]
---------+--------------------------------------------------------
    male | .0844196  .0039991                  .0765815 .0922577
  female |  .057448  .0031575                  .0512593 .0636367
---------+--------------------------------------------------------
    diff | .0269716  .0050954                  .0169849 .0369584
         | under Ho: .0050504  5.34   0.000
------------------------------------------------------------------
    diff = prop(male) - prop(female)                  z = 5.3405
 Ho: diff = 0

   Ha: diff < 0            Ha: diff != 0              Ha: diff > 0
 Pr(Z < z) = 1.0000   Pr(|Z| < |z|) = 0.0000     Pr(Z > z) = 0.0000
```

Box 7.6: Test of proportions using pull-down menus

To get to the menu for two-samples test of proportions go to:

Statistics → Summaries, tables and tests → Classical tests of hypotheses → Two-sample proportion test

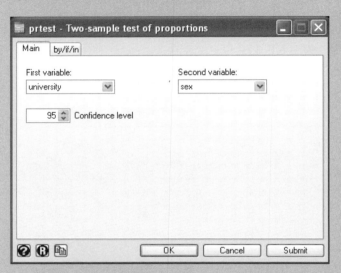

To get to the menu for a one-sample test of proportions go to:

Statistics → Summaries, tables and tests → Classical tests of hypotheses → One-sample proportion test

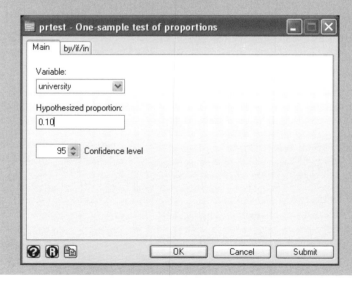

You can see that the output looks a lot like the output for an independent samples *t*-test. The **prtest** command calculates a *z* statistic and is used in a similar way to the *t* statistic. The results tell us that the null hypothesis of no difference between the proportion of males and females who have a university qualification can be rejected. There is a difference and that difference is greater than zero (i.e. more males have university qualifications).

You can also do a one-sample test of proportions in the same way that you can a one sample *t*-test. If you have some hypothesized value of a proportion which you wish to test in your data, you can set up the **prtest** in the same way you used **ttest**. Let's say, for example, that you had read a report that indicated that 10% (or 0.1 expressed as a proportion) of individuals had obtained a university qualification and you wanted to test this hypothesis in your data. You would use the command

prtest university==.10

```
. prtest university==.10

One-sample test of proportion university:    Number of obs = 10264
-----------------+----------------------------------------------------
        Variable |      Mean    Std. Err.    [95% Conf. Interval]
-----------------+----------------------------------------------------
      university |    .0701481    .0025209      .0652072    .075089
-----------------+----------------------------------------------------
 = proportion(university)                          z = -10.0811
Ho: p = 0.1

   Ha: p < 0.1              Ha: p != 0.1             Ha: p > 0.1
Pr(Z < z) = 0.0000      Pr(Z > z) = 0.0000      Pr(Z > z) = 1.0000
```

The results here indicate that the observed proportion is actually 0.07 and that this is significantly different from 0.10.

K-sample tests of proportions

There is no one agreed upon way of estimating tests of proportions for variables with more than two categories. You can obtain the different proportions by using the command **proportion** and denoting the categorical variable in parentheses after **over**.

proportion university, over(mastat)

```
. proportion university, over(mastat)

Proportion estimation                          Number of obs = 9893

      _prop_1: university = 0
      _prop_2: university = 1

      married: mastat = married
    _subpop_2: mastat = living as couple
      widowed: mastat = widowed
     divorced: mastat = divorced
    separated: mastat = separated
    _subpop_6: mastat = never married
----------+----------------------------------------------------------
          |                                          Binomial Wald
     Over | Proportion  Std. Err.    [95% Conf. Interval]
----------+----------------------------------------------------------
_prop_1   |
  married |   .9274291   .0034024    .9207597    .9340984
_subpop_2 |    .887538   .0123258     .863377     .911699
  widowed |   .9879952   .0037757    .9805941    .9953963
 divorced |   .9372093   .0117122    .9142511    .9601675
separated |   .9189189   .0201228     .879474    .9583638
_subpop_6 |   .9127789   .0063555    .9003208     .925237
----------+----------------------------------------------------------
_prop_2   |
  married |   .0725709   .0034024    .0659016    .0792403
_subpop_2 |    .112462   .0123258     .088301     .136623
  widowed |   .0120048   .0037757    .0046037    .0194059
 divorced |   .0627907   .0117122    .0398325    .0857489
separated |   .0810811   .0201228    .0416362     .120526
_subpop_6 |   .0872211   .0063555     .074763    .0996792
----------------------------------------------------------------------
```

The output here shows, by each marital status, those who do not have a university qualification, followed by those who do. There are no tests of significance for the differences of proportions, however. Significances of differences in proportions of a categorical variable can be obtained through the logistic regression estimation technique, which we will address in Chapter 8. You could also plot the proportions and their confidence intervals to determine visually if any are likely to be statistically different when their confidence intervals do not overlap.

ONE-WAY ANALYSIS OF VARIANCE

Analysis of variance (ANOVA) is an extension of the independent samples *t*-test. Instead of a dichotomous independent variable, however, your independent variable must have more than two categories. There are two commands that cover analysis of variance: **oneway** (see also Box 7.7) and **anova** (see also Box 7.8). We focus on the former as it limits the analysis to one independent variable and, as such, has many more options for what are known as 'post hoc tests'. We will return to the topic of post hoc tests shortly.

We will start with **oneway**, testing the hypothesis that there is no difference between the GHQ scale score by marital status.

oneway ghqscale mastat

```
. oneway ghqscale mastat

                      Analysis of Variance
         Source          SS    df         MS         F  Prob > F
----------------------------------------------------------------
Between groups    3808.26897     5 761.653793  32.05    0.0000
 Within groups    228313.704  9607 23.7653486
----------------------------------------------------------------
         Total    232121.973  9612 24.1491857

Bartlett's test for equal variances:    chi2(5) = 103.5783
                                     Prob>chi2 = 0.000
```

The test statistic comes from the F distribution, which, like the other distributions briefly mentioned in this book, is a distribution with its own distinct properties. Of particular relevance here is that you can find critical values of the F statistic from tables in the back of most statistics textbooks. However, Stata provides you with output that tells you that an F statistic of 32.05, with 5 and 9607 degrees of freedom, has a very low p value. In other words, there is a very low probability (less than 1 in 1000) that there are no differences in the mean *ghqscale* scores across categories of marital status. We can confidently reject the null hypothesis that there are no differences.

The final line of the output reports Bartlett's test for equality of variances. One of ANOVA's assumptions is that all the groups have equal variances. The null hypothesis for this test is that the groups have equal variances, so in this example we have to reject that hypothesis and question whether ANOVA is appropriate for this analysis. There is considerable literature on the sensitivity of Bartlett's test to any departures from normality, so it might be worth checking your data with other tests before deciding what to do. One alternative method is Levene's test within the **sdtest** command. This can only be used when you have two groups to compare across as in a t-test. Another alternative is a variation on Levene's test using robust estimations in the command **robvar**. This is not limited to two groups and so is suitable for this example.

robvar ghqscale, by(mastat)

. robvar ghqscale,by(mastat)

marital status	Summary of general health questionnaire: likert Mean	Std. Dev.	Freq.
married	10.661552	4.6695253	5670
living as	10.869565	5.0682808	644
widowed	11.777202	5.0923608	772
divorced	12.353081	6.1841094	422
separated	13.133333	6.1284208	180
never mar	10.09039	4.8560501	1925
Total	10.771247	4.9141821	9613

W0 = 13.570575 df(5, 9607)   Pr > F = 3.195e-13

W50 = 10.821274 df(5, 9607)   Pr > F = 2.133e-10

W10 = 11.579548 df(5, 9607)   Pr > F = 3.571e-11

In this case the robust tests also reject the null hypothesis of no differences as shown by the low p value (Pr). Another suggested way is to transform the interval level variable so that it is as normal as possible. In the demonstration exercise for Chapter 5 we tested transforming the *ghqscale* variable but with mixed results.

As a demonstration of the characteristics of the different tests we created a variable for three age categories (*agecat*) and tested for homogeneity of variance in the *ghqscale* variable using Levene's robust test and Bartlett's test in a one-way ANOVA:

. robvar ghqscale,by(agecat)

RECODE of age (age)	Summary of general health questionnaire: likert Mean	Std. Dev.	Freq.
1	10.427369	4.7951327	3683
2	11.09105	5.0843162	3218
3	10.858776	4.840309	2712
Total	10.771247	4.9141821	9613

W0 = 2.478514   df(2, 9610)   Pr > F = .08392137

W50 = 1.6889743   df(2, 9610)   Pr > F = .1847637

W10 = 2.3004335   df(2, 9610)   Pr > F = .10027058

```
. oneway ghqscale agecat

                      Analysis of Variance
        Source          SS      df         MS       F  Prob > F
------------------------------------------------------------------
Between groups    785.418154    2  392.709077   16.31   0.0000
 Within groups    231336.555 9610  24.0724823
------------------------------------------------------------------
       Total      232121.973 9612  24.1491857

Bartlett's test for equal variances:       chi2(2) = 13.5783
                                       Prob>chi2 = 0.000
```

As you can see, the **robvar** command results suggest that we cannot reject the null hypothesis of equal variances but the Bartlett's test in the **oneway** command suggests that we do reject the null hypothesis. Obviously we could spend considerable time on this problem, but let's continue with our examples with these variables regardless!

One thing that is very important for the novice researcher to be aware of is that this finding – that we reject the null hypothesis that there is no difference in the GHQ means for people in different marital statuses – tells us no more than that. Thus far, we do not know where those differences are. We may have an idea, for example, that those divorced or separated might have higher GHQ scores than married people. But the results from the one-way ANOVA alone do not tell us this.

If you want to see the actual means by group, then using the **ta** option after the **oneway** command produces a table of means:

oneway ghqscale mastat, ta

```
. oneway ghqscale mastat, ta

              |    Summary of general health
   marital    |      questionnaire: likert
   status     |    Mean     Std. Dev.      Freq.
--------------+---------------------------------
    married   |  10.661552   4.6695253      5670
  living as   |  10.869565   5.0682808       644
    widowed   |  11.777202   5.0923608       772
   divorced   |  12.353081   6.1841094       422
  separated   |  13.133333   6.1284208       180
  never mar   |  10.09039    4.8560501      1925
--------------+---------------------------------
      Total   |  10.771247   4.9141821      9613
```

```
                      Analysis of Variance
               Source         SS    df           MS        F  Prob > F
     ------------------------------------------------------------------
      Between groups  3808.26897     5  761.653793  32.05    0.0000
       Within groups  228313.704  9607  23.7653486
     ------------------------------------------------------------------
               Total  232121.973  9612  24.1491857

     Bartlett's test for equal variances:     chi2(5) = 103.5783
                                              Prob>chi2 = 0.000
```

Box 7.7: One-way ANOVA using pull-down menus

Go to:

**Statistics → Linear models and related → ANOVA/MANOVA →
One-way ANOVA**

and fill in the dialogue box:

Summary statistics can be obtained by ticking the **Produce
summary table** box. For Scheffé post hoc tests, you can simply
check the box under **Multiple-comparison tests** marked **Scheffe**.

Without the additional **ta** command, we only know that the means are different. With **ta** we can see what the differences *might* be. We don't know for certain, however, which groups have significant differences. The statistically significant F statistic only tells us that there is at least one difference between two means. This is where post hoc tests come into play. What we need to do next is some post hoc testing. That is, we want to compare all the means by all possible pairs of categories of marital status.

There are three post hoc tests available as options to go with the **oneway** command: **scheffe**, **sidak**, and **bonferroni**. What are the differences between these tests? There is a substantial debate in the literature about which post hoc test is most appropriate and which are the most conservative, but the Scheffé test is probably the most useful for the novice researcher because it is the only such test that is completely consistent with ANOVA results in that if the F statistic is statistically significant, then at least one of the pairs of comparisons will be significant at the same p value (Ruxton and Beauchamp 2008). In other words, if your F statistic is significant at the 0.05 level, then at least one of your pairs of means will also be significantly different from each other at this level. If you are interested in learning more about these (and other) post hoc tests used in analysis of variance, see Rutherford (2001) and Turner and Thayer (2001).

As suggested above, the **scheffe** option (Scheffé multiple comparison test) provides us with a way to determine which differences are significant. We know that there will be at least one significant difference because using **scheffe** ensures this.

oneway ghqscale mastat, scheffe

```
. oneway ghqscale mastat, scheffe

                    Analysis of Variance
        Source          SS      df        MS       F   Prob > F
------------------------------------------------------------------
Between groups     3808.26897     5 761.653793  32.05   0.0000
 Within groups     228313.704  9607 23.7653486
------------------------------------------------------------------
        Total     232121.973  9612 24.1491857

Bartlett's test for equal variances:      chi2(5) = 103.5783
                                        Prob>chi2 =  0.000
```

```
             Comparison of general health questionnaire:
                  likert by marital status (Scheffe)
Row Mean- |
Col Mean  |    married living a  widowed divorced separate
----------+-------------------------------------------------
living a  |    .208013
          |     0.958
          |
widowed   |    1.11565   .907637
          |     0.000     0.033
          |
divorced  |    1.69153   1.48352   .575878
          |     0.000     0.000     0.577
          |
separate  |    2.47178   2.26377   1.35613   .780253
          |     0.000     0.000     0.046     0.664
          |
never ma  |   -.571162  -.779176  -1.68681  -2.26269  -3.04294
          |     0.001     0.031     0.000     0.000     0.000
```

From the results, we can see that there is a significant mean difference in mental health scores between married people and all other categories apart from 'living as a couple'. The p values are shown beneath the test statistic. We can also see that there are significant differences between 'living as a couple' and being divorced, separated and never married. In fact, as we continue to go through the table there are more significant differences than non-significant ones – the majority of p values are under 0.05. It is perhaps more efficient to say that there are significant differences in mean GHQ scores between all marital statuses except between those cohabiting and married, divorced and separated, and divorced and widowed.

Box 7.8: Multivariate ANOVA

While this chapter is mostly concerned with bivariate techniques, we should also mention that multivariate analyses are possible using the **anova** command. When used with one independent variable, the **anova** command produces results that are substantively the same as **oneway**.

anova ghqscale mastat

```
. anova ghqscale mastat

      Number of obs =      9613     R-squared      = 0.0164
      Root MSE       = 4.87497     Adj R-squared  = 0.0159

    Source | Partial SS    df          MS      F  Prob > F
  ---------+--------------------------------------------------
     Model | 3808.26897     5 761.653793  32.05   0.0000
           |
    mastat | 3808.26897     5 761.653793  32.05   0.0000
           |
  Residual | 228313.704  9607 23.7653486
  ---------+--------------------------------------------------
     Total | 232121.973  9612 24.1491857
```

The **anova** command output presents additional information such as the model fit (R^2 and adjusted R^2), and sums of squares for our overall model, the independent variable, and the residual.

The main difference between **anova** and **oneway** is that **anova** allows us to add multiple independent variables. When two or more categorical independent variables are added to an analysis of variance, it is known as a factorial ANOVA.

anova ghqscale mastat sex jbstat

```
. anova ghqscale mastat sex jbstat

      Number of obs =      9613     R-squared      = 0.0711
      Root MSE       = 4.73991     Adj R-squared  = 0.0697

    Source | Partial SS    df          MS      F  Prob > F
  ---------+--------------------------------------------------
     Model | 16508.6954    15 1100.57969  48.99   0.0000
           |
    mastat | 1899.73392     5 379.946784  16.91   0.0000
       sex | 1847.50677     1 1847.50677  82.23   0.0000
    jbstat | 10644.3226     9 1182.70252  52.64   0.0000
           |
  Residual | 215613.277  9597 22.4667372
  ---------+--------------------------------------------------
     Total | 232121.973  9612 24.1491857
```

The results here show that there are differences in mean GHQ score between at least two marital status groups, between males and females, and between at least two job status groups. Again, these results do not tell you where the differences are – just that there are differences in the data. And unlike the command **oneway**, no post hoc tests are available.

In addition to analysis of variance, there is also an extension to this test called analysis of covariance (ANCOVA) in which interval predictors are added. Interval level variables must be in

▶

▶ parentheses after the **continuous** option so that Stata knows not to treat the values as nominal categories! Let's add *age* to this model, as demonstrated below.

anova ghqscale mastat sex jbstat age, continuous(age)

```
. anova ghqscale mastat sex jbstat age, continuous (age)

        Number of obs =      9613     R-squared      = 0.0711
        Root MSE      = 4.74014     Adj R-squared = 0.0696

        Source |  Partial SS    df            MS       F  Prob > F
    -----------+----------------------------------------------------
         Model |  16510.1611    16 1031.88507  45.92    0.0000
               |
        mastat |  1809.43004     5 361.886008  16.11    0.0000
           sex |  1833.15881     1 1833.15881  81.59    0.0000
        jbstat |  10618.0733     9 1179.78592  52.51    0.0000
           age |  1.46572791     1 1.46572791   0.07    0.7984
               |
      Residual |  215611.812  9596 22.4689258
    -----------+----------------------------------------------------
         Total |  232121.973  9612 24.1491857
```

Through the pull-down menus, you would go to:

Statistics → Linear models and related → ANOVA/MANOVA → Analysis of variance and covariance

You would add the variables to the dialogue box as follows:

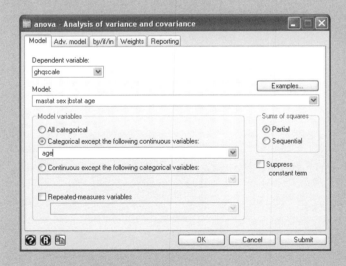

The results show that even after adjusting for age, GHQ scores still differ by marital status, sex, and job status.

You can also add interaction terms in **anova**. We will talk more about interaction terms in Chapters 8 and 9 but, basically, interaction terms test for the differential effect of an independent variable on the dependent variable, based on the value of a second independent variable. For example, we may think that mean mental health score varies by job status, but that the influence of job status will differ by sex: we may expect unemployed males to be exhibit poorer mental health than unemployed females. By placing an asterisk between the two variables of interest, we can test this assumption:

```
anova ghqscale mastat sex*jbstat
```

```
. anova ghqscale mastat sex*jbstat

      Number of obs =      9613     R-squared       = 0.0724
      Root MSE      = 4.73873     Adj R-squared = 0.0701

      Source | Partial SS    df            MS       F Prob > F
  -----------+----------------------------------------------------
       Model | 16796.0239    23 730.261907 32.52     0.0000
             |
      mastat | 1903.4685      5    380.6937 16.95     0.0000
  sex*jbstat | 12987.7549    18 721.541939 32.13     0.0000
             |
    Residual | 215325.949  9589 22.4555166
  -----------+----------------------------------------------------
       Total |  232121.973  9612 24.1491857
```

To add an interaction in the dialogue box, just put an asterisk between the two variables you wish to interact.

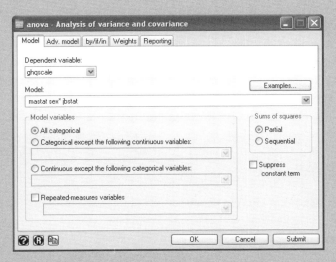

The results here confirm that there is a statistically significant interaction between sex and job status – therefore, the mean GHQ score of men and women varies by job status.

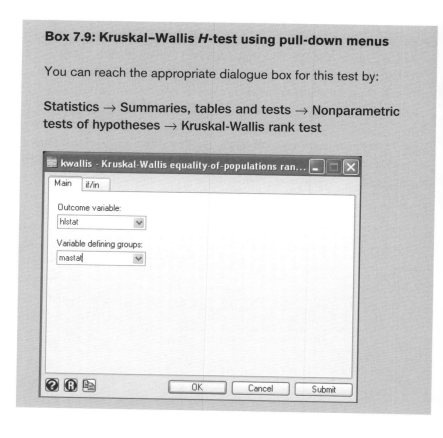

> **Box 7.9: Kruskal–Wallis *H*-test using pull-down menus**
>
> You can reach the appropriate dialogue box for this test by:
>
> Statistics → Summaries, tables and tests → Nonparametric
> tests of hypotheses → Kruskal-Wallis rank test

Kruskal–Wallis *H*-test

The Kruskal–Wallis *H*-test is the non-parametric alternative to the
one-way analysis of variance (see also Box 7.9). It allows you to
compare the scores on some ordinal variable for three or more
groups. Scores are converted to ranks, and the mean rank for each
group is compared. This is a 'between groups' analysis, and therefore different people must be in each of the different groups. Let's
examine whether the ordinal variable health status (*hlstat*) differs
by marital status.

kwallis hlstat, by(mastat)

```
. kwallis hlstat, by(mastat)

Test: Equality of populations (Kruskal-Wallis
test)
```

```
+----------------------------------------+
|  mastat  |    Obs  |    Rank Sum  |
+----------+---------+---------------+
|  married |   6007  |    3.04e+07  |
| living a |    673  |    3.31e+06  |
|  widowed |    862  |    5.31e+06  |
| divorced |    433  |    2.38e+06  |
| separate |    189  |    1.05e+06  |
+----------+---------+---------------+
| never ma |   2092  |    1.01e+07  |
+----------------------------------------+
```

chi-squared = 142.776 with 5 d.f.
probability =   0.0001

chi-squared with ties = 162.331 with 5 d.f.
probability   = 0.0001

The results above report the number of observations and the sum of the ranks. Because the sample sizes here are very large, the rank sums are expressed in exponential terms – for example, the rank sum for married is expressed as 3.04e+07, which is equivalent to 30,400,000. There are two chi-squared values reported – one without ties and one with ties. If there were 'ties' between some of the scores (i.e., they ended up in the same 'rank'), then a 'correction factor' is included in the chi-squared statistic. However, whether or not a correction for ties is taken into account, the results are statistically significant – the average score on self-reported health status differs by marital status. For a practical application of tests for differences between groups, see Box 7.10.

REPEATED MEASURES

This chapter has focused on cross-sectional tests – that is, examining the midpoint value of a variable at one point in time across groups. In many cases, however, researchers are interested in comparing scores over time. This is where repeated measures tests come in. In this section, we discuss the repeated measure equivalents of the tests already discussed. It should be noted that there are no directly equivalent repeated measures tests for the tests of proportions.

Box 7.10: Using one-way ANOVA and Kruskal–Wallis tests in an applied research project

In a study[1] of the effectiveness of three different cleaning protocols in isolation wards we were faced with the problem of analysing two main outcome measures of bacterial counts from various locations in the wards. The first outcome was a count of methicillin-resistant *Staphylococcus aureus* (MRSA) and the second outcome was total viable bacterial counts (TVCs). The MRSA count data were highly skewed as many of the sites had zero counts. In order to test if the counts varied between cleaning methods we used a non-parametric test. As we had three cleaning methods we used a Kruskal–Wallis test. The outcome measure was the MRSA count and the factor was the cleaning method variable. The TVCs data were a little more problematic as they were an interval level measure and for some of the sites their distribution was reasonably normally distributed, whereas in other sites it was somewhat skewed. Preliminary analysis showed that there were some extreme outliers and they were driving apparent differences in means. Therefore, we transformed the TVCs data using the base 10 logarithm and reported both the raw and transformed means and standard deviations in the table, although the one-way ANOVA and post hoc Bonferroni tests were only done on the transformed data.

[1] Patel, S.S., Pevalin, D.J., Prosser, R. and Couchman, A. (2007) Comparison of detergent-based cleaning, disinfectant-based cleaning, and detergent-based cleaning after enhanced domestic staff training within a source isolation facility. *British Journal of Infection Control* 8(3): 20–25.

Paired *t*-tests

Paired *t*-tests compute their findings on paired observations, so if an observation is missing for a person, that person is eliminated from the test. You would do a paired *t*-test, for example, if you wanted to compare respondents' scores on an item from one year to the next. This test is sometimes called a repeated measures *t*-test. The data need to be in wide format (see Chapter 4).

Suppose you wanted to test whether the mean GHQ score was the same for individuals in two successive years. The variable measuring GHQ in the 1991 is called *ghq91* and in 1992 it is called *ghq92*. With a paired *t*-test, you would do this by:

```
ttest ghq91==ghq92

. ttest ghq91==ghq92

Paired t test
------------------------------------------------------------------------
Variable |  Obs       Mean   Std. Err.  Std. Dev.  [95% Conf. Interval]
---------+--------------------------------------------------------------
   ghq91 |  556    9.611511   .1074406   2.533411   9.400471   9.822551
   ghq92 |  556   11.44245    .1799025   4.242037   11.08907   11.79582
---------+--------------------------------------------------------------
    diff |  556   -1.830935   .1791348   4.223936   -2.1828    -1.47907
------------------------------------------------------------------------
    mean(diff) = mean(ghq91 - ghq92)                    t = -10.2210
Ho: mean(diff) = 0                          degrees of freedom = 555

Ha: mean(diff) < 0        Ha: mean(diff) != 0        Ha: mean(diff) > 0
Pr(T < t) = 0.0000     Pr(|T| > |t|) = 0.0000      Pr(T > t) = 1.0000
```

You can see that the mean difference between the two years was −1.831, meaning that there had been an overall increase in the GHQ score in our sample over the two years in question. The interpretations of the *t* and *p* values are the same as in the independent two-samples *t*-test. In this example, the *t* value is −10.22 with *p* = 0.0000 for a two-sided test, meaning we can reject the null hypothesis that the scores are equal for 1991 and 1992 (see also Box 7.11).

Equality tests on matched data

There are two similar tests that are non-parametric alternatives to the repeated measures (paired) *t*-test. Both are designed for use with repeated measures: that is, when your subjects are measured on two occasions, or under two different conditions. As for paired *t*-tests, the data need to be in wide format.

The two tests differ in their basic assumption. The **signrank** test is used when there is an assumption that the difference between two variables is ordinal, but there is *no assumption* that the difference between the two variables is both interval in nature and normally distributed. The alternative, **signtest**, assumes that the difference between the two variables in question is not necessarily ordinal, but merely positive or negative. Furthermore, **signtest** tests the null hypothesis that the median of the difference is zero, while **signrank** tests the null hypothesis that both distributions are the same.

Box 7.11: Repeated measures *t*-test using pull-down menus

You can reach the appropriate dialogue box for a paired *t*-test by:

Statistics → Summaries, tables and tests → Classical tests of hypotheses → Mean-comparison test, paired data

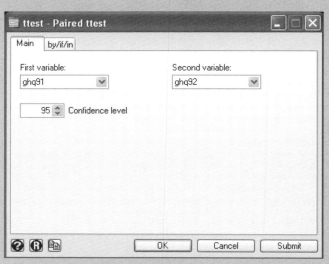

You can reach the appropriate dialogue box for the Wilcoxon signed rank test by:

Statistics → Summaries, tables and tests → Nonparametric tests of hypotheses → Wilcoxon matched-pairs signed-rank test

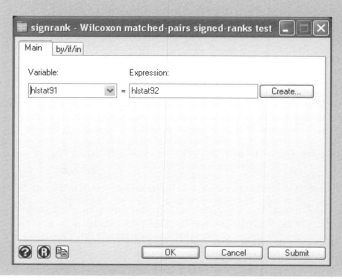

You can find the associated drop-down menu for the **signtest** command through:

Statistics → Summaries, tables and tests → Nonparametric tests of hypotheses → Test of equality of matched pairs

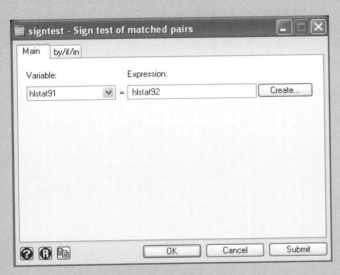

Repeated measures ANOVA can be done through the pull-down menu at:

Statistics → Linear models and related → ANOVA/MANOVA → Analysis of variance and covariance

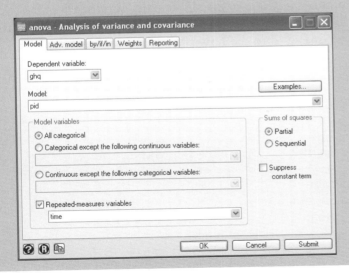

The Wilcoxon signed rank test is designed for use with repeated measures, but instead of comparing means the Wilcoxon test converts scores to ranks and compares them at time 1 and time 2. In this example we examine self-reported health status (*hlstat91* and *hlstat92*) in two successive years.

signrank hlstat91=hlstat92

```
. signrank hlstat91=hlstat92

Wilcoxon signed-rank test

        sign |      obs    sum ranks    expected
-------------+----------------------------------
    positive |      125      52710.5       54998
    negative |      132      57285.5       54998
        zero |      299        44850       44850
-------------+----------------------------------
         all |      556       154846      154846

unadjusted variance       14361967
adjustment for ties     -199398.25
adjustment for zeros   -2238762.5
                        ----------
adjusted variance         11923806

Ho: hlstat91 = hlstat92
            z =  -0.662
  Prob > |z| =  0.5077
```

The results here suggest that we cannot reject the null hypothesis of no difference, so there is no statistically significant difference between health status in 1991 and 1992. Now we can try the **signtest** command to see how our results compare.

signtest hlstat91=hlstat92

```
. signtest hlstat91= hlstat92

Sign test

        sign |    observed    expected
-------------+------------------------
    positive |         125       128.5
    negative |         132       128.5
        zero |         299         299
-------------+------------------------
         all |         556         556
```

One-sided tests:
  Ho: median of hlstat91 - hlstat92 = 0 vs.
  Ha: median of hlstat91 - bhlstat92 > 0
     Pr(#positive >= 125) =
       Binomial(n = 257, x >= 125, p = 0.5)
       = 0.6911

  Ho: median of hlstat91 - hlstat92 = 0 vs.
  Ha: median of hlstat91 - hlstat92 < 0
     Pr(#negative >= 132) =
     Binomial(n = 257, x >= 132, p = 0.5)
      = 0.3541

Two-sided test:
  Ho: median of hlstat91 - hlstat92 = 0 vs.
  Ha: median of hlstat91 - hlstat92 != 0
     Pr(#positive >= 132 or #negative >= 132)
      = min(1, 2*Binomial(n = 257, x >= 132,
      p = 0.5)) = 0.7083

The output above gives us the one-sided and two-sided tests. Because we are looking for any difference (i.e. we did not hypothesize the direction of the difference), we would look to the two-sided test and conclude that no statistically significant difference was found as $p = 0.708$.

Repeated measures analysis of variance

Repeated measures analysis of variance is done using the **anova** command with the option **repeated**. You would use repeated measures ANOVA if you had an interval level dependent variable and one categorical independent variable which was repeated at least once (i.e. there were two observations for each individual). This test is an extension of the paired samples t-test in that you can have an independent variable with more than two categories. It should be emphasized that the test also works for independent variables with two categories as well.

A major difference between repeated measures ANOVA and the other tests discussed so far is that this technique requires that your data be in long file format. We haven't analysed data in long file format yet in this book. If you recall from Chapter 4, long file format is when all your cases are stacked on top of each other by time of observation, with an additional variable denoting the time. So an individual would have separate rows in the spreadsheet at time 1 and time 2.

We have been working with data in wide format. In the example below, *pid* is the individual personal identifier, *ghq1* is the GHQ score in the first year, *ghq2* is the GHQ score in the second year and *ghq3* is the GHQ score in the third year:

pid	ghq1	ghq2	ghq3
1	11	22	8
2	6	8	10
3	11	9	10

In order to look at GHQ scores over multiple years using repeated measures ANOVA, we would need the data to be set up as follows:

pid	time	ghq
1	1	11
1	2	22
1	3	8
2	1	6
2	2	8
2	3	10
3	1	11
3	2	9
3	3	10

We can convert the data from wide file format into long file format with the command:

```
reshape ghq time pid, repeated(time)
```

The **reshape** command is quite advanced but more fully described in Chapter 4.

Now we can see whether the mean GHQ score varies by time using the **anova** command.

anova ghq time pid, repeated(time)

```
. anova ghq time pid, repeated(time)

          Number of obs =   1629        R-squared = 0.4954
                  Root MSE = 4.048   Adj R-squared = 0.2330

   Source | Partial SS    df            MS       F    Prob > F
---------+-----------------------------------------------------
   Model | 17234.2065   557    30.9411248   1.89    0.0000
         |
    time | 1163.21909     2    581.609546 35.48    0.0000
     pid | 16071.0669   555    28.9568772  1.77    0.0000
         |
Residual | 17554.9476  1071    16.3911742
---------+-----------------------------------------------------
   Total | 34789.1541  1628    21.3692593

Between-subjects error term: pid
Levels:                           556        (555 df)
Lowest b.s.e. variable:           pid

Repeated variable: time
                          Huynh-Feldt epsilon = 0.8089
                   Greenhouse-Geisser epsilon = 0.8069
                   Box's conservative epsilon = 0.5000

                          ------- Prob > F ------
   Source |       df      F Regular    H-F     G-G     Box
---------+-----------------------------------------------------
    time |      2 35.48   0.0000 0.0000 0.0000 0.0000
Residual |   1071
---------+-----------------------------------------------------
```

The output tells us that the F statistic (35.48) for the variable *time* is statistically significant ($p = 0.000$). The output gives us three additional p value measures: H-F corresponds to the Huynh–Feldt G-G to the Greenhouse–Geisser, and Box to Box's conservative p-value. However, no matter which p value you choose, the results are significant at the 0.05 level. For more information on the different types of p values associated with repeated measures ANOVA, see Cardinal and Aitken (2006).

Friedman test

The Friedman test is a non-parametric version of repeated measures ANOVA. You would perform this test when your independent variable has more than two categories and your dependent variable is at the ordinal level of measurement. We will use this test to determine if there is a difference in the self-reported health status of individuals over three years of the data. The null hypothesis in this test is that the distribution of the ranks of each type of score (i.e. *hlstat1*, *hlstat2*, and *hlstat3*) is the same.

To conduct the Friedman test, you need to download and install the **friedman** program. It is not available in Stata as a default program (at the time of writing). To install **friedman** type

findit friedman

and follow the prompts for installation. Note that your computer must be connected to the internet for this to work! Because the program is not built into Stata, there are no drop-down menus for it.

Like the repeated measures ANOVA, we must transform the data somewhat before we can use the **friedman** command. Currently, our data are in wide format and look like this:

pid	*hlstat1*	*hlstat2*	*hlstat3*
1	2	2	1
2	3	1	5
3	2	2	2
4	4	5	2
5	3	3	2
6	2	3	3

Here *pid* is the personal identification number, *hlstat1* is self reported health status in year 1, *hlstat2* is self-reported health status in year 2 and *hlstat3* is self-reported health status in year 3. The Friedman test requires that our data take a 'transposed' shape, which is neither 'wide' nor 'long'. Essentially, our data must look like this:

pers1	pers2	pers3	pers4	pers5	pers6
2	3	2	4	3	2
2	1	2	5	3	3
1	5	2	2	2	3

Here *pers* variables are individuals' scores for each of the three years.

To get the data into this shape, we need to first keep only the variables (be sure to save your data set beforehand!).

```
keep hlstat1 hlstat2 hlstat3
```

We also must drop any cases with missing values. This is because the **friedman** command cannot be computed if there is even one missing value. You will get an error. So before we go any further, it is necessary to deal with missing cases.

```
drop if hlstat1==.|hlstat2==.|hlstat3==.
```

Then we use the command **xpose** which transposes all variables into observations and observations into variables.

```
xpose, clear
```

After performing the **xpose** command, you will see that the data have been transformed into numerous variables – in fact, as many variables as there are cases in the data. So, before using **xpose** the variable window will look like this:

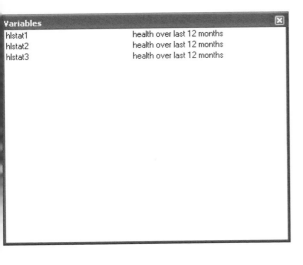

After using **xpose** it will look like this:

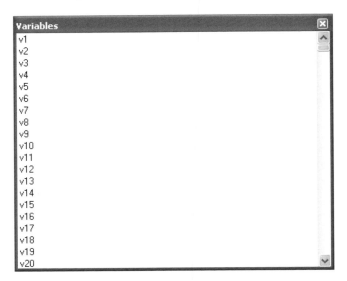

If you scroll down, you can see that each person has become a variable in the data set.

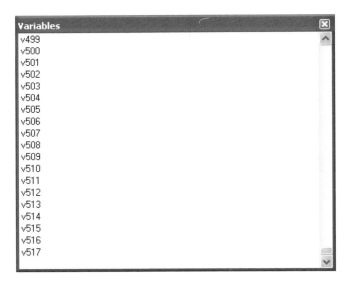

Now we are ready to perform the Friedman test.

friedman v1-v517

```
. friedman v1-v517

Friedman = 2.8849
Kendall  = 0.0028
p-value  = 0.2363
```

We type **v1-v517** because we have 517 variables in our data set.
Friedman's chi-square is reported as 2.885 with a *p* value of 0.236
and is therefore not statistically significant. Hence, there is no
evidence that the distributions of the variable are different at the
three time points.

DEMONSTRATION EXERCISE

In Chapter 3 we manipulated the individual level variables and
saved a new data set called demodata1.dta. In Chapter 4 we
merged a household level variable indicating the region of the
country onto the individual level data and saved the data with a
new name demodata2.dta. In Chapter 5 we examined the variables we are using for their distribution, measures of central tendency and, for continuous variables, their normality. In Chapter 6
we examined differences in mean GHQ scale scores across groups
in the factors but did not formally test for differences. The
dichotomous indicator was tested using the **tab** command and
measures of association. Correlations between the GHQ scale and
interval level factors were produced.

At this stage of the demonstration we test for differences
in mean GHQ (*ghqscale*) scores across groups of the categorical
factors using **ttest** and **oneway** commands.

Let's start with the *t*-tests. The only dichotomous factor is
the *female* variable. First we need to determine if there are equal
variances in the *ghqscale* variable across the groups of the *female*
variable. Here, we use Levene's test:

ttest ghqscale,by(female)

```
sdtest ghqscale,by(female)

Variance ratio test

------------------------------------------------------------------------
  Group |    Obs       Mean   Std. Err.   Std. Dev.   [95% Conf. Interval]
--------+---------------------------------------------------------------
   male |   3645   10.1668    .0792765    4.786225    10.01137   10.32223
 female |   4069  11.29909    .0799825    5.101984    11.14228    11.4559
--------+---------------------------------------------------------------
combined |  7714  10.76407    .0567819    4.987117    10.65276   10.87537
------------------------------------------------------------------------
   ratio = sd(male) / sd(female)                         f = 0.8801
Ho: ratio = 1                              degrees of freedom = 3644, 4068

Ha: ratio < 1             Ha: ratio != 1                Ha: ratio > 1
Pr(F < f) = 0.0000      2*Pr(F < f) = 0.0001          Pr(F > f) = 1.0000
```

Examining the output from Levene's test, you can see that the probability for the two-tail test under the `Ha: ratio != 1` hypothesis is less than 0.01. In which case, we must reject the hypothesis that the groups have equal variances. The **ttest** command thus needs to use the **unequal** option:

ttest ghqscale, by(female) unequal

```
. ttest ghqscale, by(female) unequal

Two-sample t test with unequal variances
------------------------------------------------------------------------------
   Group |     Obs       Mean   Std. Err.   Std. Dev.   [95% Conf. Interval]
---------+--------------------------------------------------------------------
    male |    3645    10.1668   .0792765    4.786225    10.01137   10.3222
  female |    4069   11.29909   .0799825    5.101984    11.14228   11.455
---------+--------------------------------------------------------------------
combined |    7714   10.76407   .0567819    4.987117    10.65276   10.8753
---------+--------------------------------------------------------------------
    diff |           -1.132287   .1126142               -1.353041 -.911532
------------------------------------------------------------------------------
    diff = mean(male) - mean(female)                          t = -10.054
Ho: diff = 0               Satterthwaite's degrees of freedom =   7695.5

   Ha: diff < 0              Ha: diff != 0               Ha: diff > 0
Pr(T < t) = 0.0000    Pr(|T| > |t|) = 0.0000        Pr(T > t) = 1.000
```

These results indicate that, on average, females have higher GHQ scores.

Next, let's turn to one-way ANOVAs to test for difference across the other categorical variables. We run all five in one go in a do file:

oneway ghqscale agecat
oneway ghqscale marst2
oneway ghqscale empstat
oneway ghqscale numchd
oneway ghqscale region2

```
. oneway ghqscale agecat

                        Analysis of Variance
        Source              SS      df       MS       F  Prob >
-------------------------------------------------------------------
Between groups        361.63595     2  180.817975  7.28    0.000
 Within groups       191470.963  7711  24.8308861
-------------------------------------------------------------------
        Total       191832.599  7713   24.871334

Bartlett's test for equal variances:          chi2(2) = 0.889
                                           Prob>chi2 = 0.641
```

. oneway ghqscale marst2

```
                     Analysis of Variance
          Source            SS     df         MS        F  Prob > F
-------------------------------------------------------------------
Between groups    2579.52626     3 859.842085  35.03     0.0000
 Within groups    189253.073  7710 24.5464426
-------------------------------------------------------------------
       Total    191832.599  7713   24.871334

Bartlett's test for equal variances:     chi2(3) = 102.9482
                                         Prob>chi2 = 0.000
```

. oneway ghqscale empstat

```
                     Analysis of Variance
          Source            SS     df         MS        F  Prob > F
-------------------------------------------------------------------
Between groups    10625.9638     5 2125.19276  90.60     0.0000
 Within groups    180191.602  7682 23.4563398
-------------------------------------------------------------------
       Total    190817.566  7687 24.8234117

Bartlett's test for equal variances:     chi2(5) = 261.5291
                                         Prob>chi2 = 0.000
```

. oneway ghqscale numchd

```
                     Analysis of Variance
          Source            SS     df         MS        F  Prob > F
-------------------------------------------------------------------
Between groups    733.106038     2 366.553019  14.79     0.0000
 Within groups    191099.493  7711 24.7827121
-------------------------------------------------------------------
       Total    191832.599  7713   24.871334

Bartlett's test for equal variances:     chi2(2) = 1.0408
                                         Prob>chi2 = 0.594
```

. oneway ghqscale region2

```
                     Analysis of Variance
          Source            SS     df         MS        F  Prob > F
-------------------------------------------------------------------
Between groups    365.691798     6 60.9486331   2.45     0.0226
 Within groups    191466.907  7707 24.8432473
-------------------------------------------------------------------
       Total    191832.599  7713   24.871334

Bartlett's test for equal variances:     chi2(6) = 37.9847
                                         Prob>chi2 = 0.000
```

The *F* statistics are significant ($p < 0.05$) for all categorical vari
ables. However, the Barlett tests indicate that there might be
some issues of unequal variance across the groups for the factors
empstat, *marst2* and *region2*. As we mentioned earlier in this
chapter, Bartlett's test can be sensitive to minor departures from
normality, so we will use the robust Levene test in the **robvar**
command to further investigate the variances.

```
robvar ghqscale,by(empstat)
robvar ghqscale,by(marst2)
robvar ghqscale,by(region2)
```

. robvar ghqscale,by(empstat)

employment status	Summary of ghq 0-36		
	Mean	Std. Dev.	Freq.
employed	10.228535	4.457344	5474
unemploye	12.910569	6.1352816	492
longterm	15.348936	6.8884231	235
studying	10.343891	5.1185333	221
family ca	12.105562	5.654763	881
retired	10	4.5546451	385
Total	10.763658	4.9823099	7688

W0 = 40.243034 df(6, 7707)   Pr > F = 1.644e-48

W50 = 32.036602 df(6, 7707)   Pr > F = 2.658e-38

W10 = 35.719273 df(6, 7707)   Pr > F = 6.933e-43

. robvar ghqscale,by(marst2)

marital status 4 categories	Summary of ghq 0-36		
	Mean	Std. Dev.	Freq.
single	10.300135	5.0855403	1486
married	10.661094	4.7401956	5503
sep/div	12.601818	6.2950812	550
widowed	12.165714	5.603875	175
Total	10.764065	4.9871168	7714

W0 = 22.673672 df(3, 7710)   Pr > F = 1.309e-14

W50 = 18.096946 df(3, 7710)   Pr > F = 1.066e-11

W10 = 19.602513 df(3, 7710)   Pr > F = 1.177e-12

```
. robvar ghqscale,by(region2)
```

regions 7 categories	Summary of ghq 0-36		
	Mean	Std. Dev.	Freq.
London	10.886169	5.2436252	817
South	10.595925	4.6873965	2356
Midlands	10.767092	5.1124056	1331
Northwest	10.722222	4.8574869	810
North and	10.806555	5.0410464	1251
Wales	11.600503	5.6429176	398
Scotland	10.684421	5.0372225	751
Total	10.764065	4.9871168	7714

```
W0  = 3.9171877 df(6, 7707)   Pr > F = .00065247

W50 = 2.7382873 df(6, 7707)   Pr > F = .01168475

W10 = 3.134685  df(6, 7707)   Pr > F = .00453326
```

The Levene tests indicate that there are significant differences in variance across the groups of these three factors. At this point it is worth considering transforming the interval level variable. We used a natural log transformation to see if this would help reduce the differences in variance across the groups:

gen lnghq=ln(ghqscale)

Then we used the **robvar** command again, but this time with the new *lnghq* variable. Significant differences in variance remained in the *empstat* and *marst2* factors, but the transformation reduced the differences in the *region2* factor to the extent that we did not reject the null hypothesis of no differences. At this point we should now be cautious of our ANOVA results for the *empstat* and *marst2* factors.

In Chapter 6 we used two-way tables and measures of association to examine whether the dichotomous GHQ indicator (*d_ghq*) had any statistical associations with the categorical factors. In this chapter we can test for a difference of proportions across gender using the **prtest** command.

prtest d_ghq,by(female)

```
. prtest d_ghq,by(female)

Two-sample test of proportion              male: Number of obs = 3645
                                         female: Number of obs = 4069
--------------------------------------------------------------------
   Variable |     Mean  Std. Err.     z  P>|z|   [95% Conf. Interval]
------------+-------------------------------------------------------
       male |  .1632373  .0061216                 .1512393  .1752353
     female |   .208405  .0063674                 .1959251  .2208849
------------+-------------------------------------------------------
       diff | -.0451677  .0088327                -.0624795 -.0278559
            | under Ho:  .0088934 -5.08 0.000
--------------------------------------------------------------------
       diff = prop(male) - prop(female)                   z = -5.0788
   Ho: diff = 0

Ha: diff < 0                  Ha: diff != 0                  Ha: diff > 0
Pr(Z < z) = 0.0000    Pr(|Z| < |z|) = 0.0000      Pr(Z > z) = 1.0000
```

If you refer back to Chapter 6 then you will see that when we used
a chi-squared test on a two-way table of *d_ghq* and *female* we got
the following result:

```
ta d_ghq female, chi2 nofreq
        Pearson chi2(1) = 25.7939   Pr = 0.000
```

Thus, the test of proportions supports the previous results. At this
point we could use the proportion command to see the distribution of the *d_ghq* variable over the other categorical variables, but
this would not give any more information than we could get with
a table and the table has the advantage of producing a measure of
association. For demonstration:

ta marst2 d_ghq, row chi2 nokey nofreq
proportion d_ghq,over(marst2)

If you compare the shaded results from the two-way table and
the shaded results from the **proportion** command you can see
that you obtain the same information but the chi-squared statistic
for the table tells you that there is a significant association.
Sometimes the simplest approach gives you all the information
you need!

```
. ta marst2 d_ghq , row chi2 nokey nofreq

   marital |
  status 4 |      d_ghq
categories |       0          1 |     Total
-----------+-----------------+---------
    single |    82.23     17.77 |    100.00
   married |    82.32     17.68 |    100.00
   sep/div |    70.00     30.00 |    100.00
   widowed |    76.57     23.43 |    100.00
-----------+-----------------+---------
     Total |    81.29     18.71 |    100.00

         Pearson chi2(3) = 53.3636   Pr = 0.000

. proportion d_ghq,over(marst2)

Proportion estimation                Number of obs = 7714

    _prop_1: d_ghq = 0
    _prop_2: d_ghq = 1

    single: marst2 = single
   married: marst2 = married
 _subpop_3: marst2 = sep/div
   widowed: marst2 = widowed

-----------------------------------------------------------
           |                      Binomial Wald
      Over | Proportion  Std. Err.  [95% conf. Interval]
-----------+-----------------------------------------------
_prop_1    |
    single |   .8223419   .0099187   .8028985  .8417852
   married |   .8231874   .0051433    .813105  .8332697
 _subpop_3 |         .7    .019558   .6616611  .7383389
   widowed |   .7657143   .0321094   .7027712  .8286574
-----------+-----------------------------------------------
_prop_2    |
    single |   .1776581   .0099187   .1582148  .1971015
   married |   .1768126   .0051433   .1667303   .186895
 _subpop_3 |         .3    .019558   .2616611  .3383389
   widowed |   .2342857   .0321094   .1713426  .2972288
-----------------------------------------------------------
```

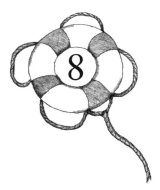

Regression

In this chapter we tackle how to conduct regression analyses in Stata. We concentrate on ordinary least squares (OLS) regression, which requires a reasonably normally distributed, interval level dependent variable, and logistic regression, which requires a dichotomous or binary dependent variable. We briefly introduce commands for multinomial logistic and ordered logistic regression models, the parallel family of commands for binary, multinomial and ordered probit, and Poisson or negative binomial models for a count dependent variable (see Box 8.1).

Among all of this we also look at the characteristics and effects of the independent variables. The majority of these techniques can be used on independent variables in any of the regression models mentioned above with more or less ease of interpretation. We will also discuss ways of dealing with categorical independent variables, non-linear associations, interaction effects, as well as regression diagnostics.

ORDINARY LEAST SQUARES REGRESSION

To carry out a bivariate regression use the **regress** (or **reg** command, immediately followed by the Y (dependent) variable and the X (independent) variable.

regress Y X

There are a number of variables in the example data set that are suitable for regression. In this example we will use monthly income (*fimn*) as our dependent variable, but considering only those in paid employment. We could use an **if** statement so that our regressions are only done where **jbstat==2**. Another way would be use a **keep** command so that only those people in employment

Box 8.1: Characteristics of dependent variables and choosing regression models

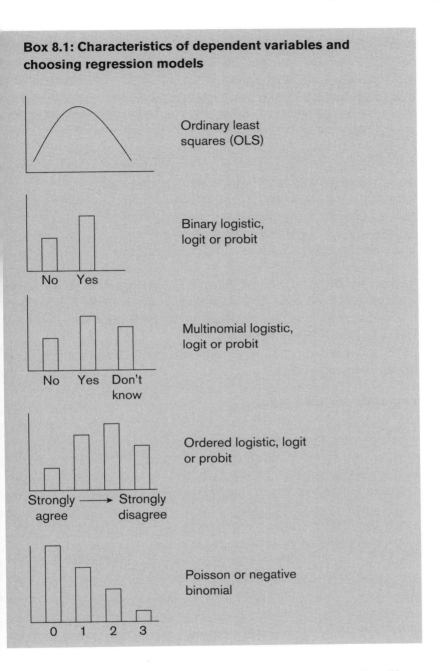

Ordinary least squares (OLS)

Binary logistic, logit or probit

No   Yes

Multinomial logistic, logit or probit

No   Yes   Don't know

Ordered logistic, logit or probit

Strongly ⟶ Strongly
agree   disagree

Poisson or negative binomial

0   1   2   3

are kept in the active data set: **keep if jbstat==2**. We will use the latter.

It is usual for income distributions to be positively skewed (or skewed to the right), in which case a natural logarithm transformation usually helps to bring the distribution closer to normality. As we have done before in Chapter 5, we can check the skewness of the original income variable and the transformed variable:

```
gen ln_inc=ln(fimn)
tabstat fimn ln_inc, s(sk kur)
```

```
. gen ln_inc=ln(fimn)

. tabstat fimn ln_inc,s(sk kur)

    stats |         fimn        ln_inc
----------+----------------------------
 skewness |     2.473931     -.5381867
 kurtosis |    18.37824      3.587047
----------+----------------------------
```

We can see from the output that the skewness and kurtosis of the variable has been considerably reduced and brought much closer to normality by the transformation. We will now use the *ln_inc* variable as our dependent variable.

First, we will use a bivariate regression to see if age is a significant determinant of income.

regress ln_inc age

```
. reg ln_inc age

    Source |       SS       df       MS              Number of obs =     497
-----------+------------------------------           F( 1,  4971) =    44.9
     Model | 21.1283285        1 21.1283285          Prob > F      = 0.000
  Residual | 2336.13556     4971 .469952838          R-squared     = 0.009
-----------+------------------------------           Adj R-squared = 0.008
     Total | 2357.26389     4972 .474107781          Root MSE      = .6855

------------------------------------------------------------------------------
    ln_inc |     Coef.  Std. Err.      t    P>|t|     [95% Conf. Interval
-----------+------------------------------------------------------------------
       age |  .0052946  .0007896    6.71   0.000     .0037465     .006842
     _cons |  6.517582  .0313587  207.84   0.000     6.456105     6.57905
------------------------------------------------------------------------------
```

The regression output is relatively concise; check the equivalent output in SPSS if you don't believe us. In the upper right-hand side is the information concerning the number of observations used in the model as the **regress** command uses listwise deletion (i.e. only cases with non-missing values on all the variables in the model will be included) and model 'fit' statistics. The most commonly used 'fit' statistic in OLS regression is R^2 (R-squared on the output

This indicates the amount of variance in the dependent variable explained by the independent variables; the higher the value, the more explanatory power the model has generally. Also in the upper right-hand corner are an F statistic and its associated p value, which becomes more useful when you are working with nested models or adding blocks of independent variables. At this stage, we suggest you do not to concern yourself with the adjusted R^2 and mean squared error statistics (`Adj R-squared` and `Root MSE` respectively on the output). The upper left-hand side of the output presents the sums of squares details as you would get from ANOVA. The lower panel of the output shows the regression coefficients, standard errors, t values, p values and 95% confidence intervals of those coefficients in each row. The bottom row starting with `_cons` is the intercept or constant for the model.

We see that even though the coefficient for age is 0.005 and is significant ($t = 6.71$ and $p = 0.000$) this isn't a very good model (bivariate models often are not), as the R^2 value is very low at 0.009 – less than 1%. It may be that the association between the dependent variable and the independent variable is not linear. Previous research informs us that age often has a curvilinear relationship with income in that income initially increases with age and then decreases. We can check if this is the case in these data with a scatterplot with *age* as the X variable and *ln_inc* as the Y variable.

scatter ln_inc age

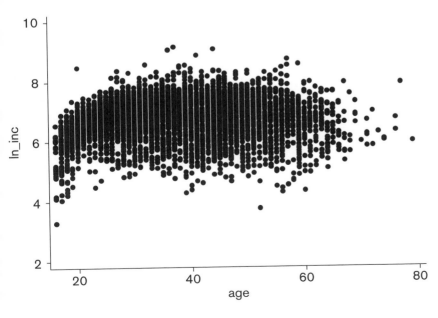

Capturing this type of non-linear association often requires the addition of a squared term of the independent variable.

gen agesq=age*age

or

gen agesq=age^2

If we rerun our regression with the transformed income variable and the *age* variable plus its square we see that our model fits much better; R^2 is now 0.067 (6.7%). The significance of the age terms (*age* and *agesq*) tells us that we were correct to assume a curvilinear relationship.

regress ln_inc age agesq

```
. reg ln_inc age agesq

    Source |       SS       df       MS              Number of obs =    4973
-----------+------------------------------           F( 2, 4970)   =  180.02
     Model | 159.233417      2  79.6167087           Prob > F      =  0.0000
  Residual | 2198.03047   4970  .442259652           R-squared     =  0.0676
-----------+------------------------------           Adj R-squared =  0.0672
     Total | 2357.26389   4972  .474107781           Root MSE      =  .66503

------------------------------------------------------------------------------
    ln_inc |      Coef.   Std. Err.      t    P>|t|     [95% Conf. Interval]
-----------+------------------------------------------------------------------
       age |   .0841962   .0045302    18.59   0.000     .0753149    .0930774
     agesq |  -.0009989   .0000565   -17.67   0.000    -.0011097   -.000888
     _cons |   5.113853   .0850617    60.12   0.000     4.947095    5.280612
------------------------------------------------------------------------------
```

We can now add some additional predictors of income to our model. First we add a variable for gender. The current variable *sex* is coded 1 = male and 2 = female. We can either recode this to a dummy variable (0,1) for either males or females or use the **xi** command (see also Box 8.2). If we prefix the **regress** command with **xi:** and putting an **i.** in front of our categorical variables of interest, Stata automatically converts them to dummy variables in our regression equation. **xi** expands terms containing categorical variables into indicator (also called dummy) variable sets by creating new variables and then executes the specified command with the expanded terms.

xi:regress ln_inc age agesq i.sex

```
. xi:reg ln_inc age agesq i.sex
i.sex         _Isex_1-2        (naturally coded; _Isex_1 omitted)
```

Source	SS	df	MS		Number of obs =	4973
					F(3, 4969) =	641.84
Model	658.344919	3	219.448306		Prob > F =	0.0000
Residual	1698.91897	4969	.341903596		R-squared =	0.2793
					Adj R-squared =	0.2788
Total	2357.26389	4972	.474107781		Root MSE =	.58473

ln_inc	Coef.	Std. Err.	t	P>|t|	[95% Conf.	Interval]
age	.0905245	.0039866	22.71	0.000	.0827089	.09834
agesq	-.0010799	.0000497	-21.71	0.000	-.0011774	-.0009824
_Isex_2	-.6342055	.016599	-38.21	0.000	-.6667469	-.601664
_cons	5.322339	.0749894	70.97	0.000	5.175327	5.469352

Note that at the bottom of the variable list a new variable (_Isex_2) has appeared. This is the dummy variable automatically created by Stata for the original variable *sex*. The output line immediately after the command shows how Stata has created dummy or indicator variables out of the *sex* variable:

```
i.sex  _Isex_1-2  (naturally coded; _Isex_1 omitted)
```

This line shows at the left that the variable *sex* was indicated with an **i.** prefix in the command line. The next part (_Isex_1-2) shows that indicator variables have been created (_I) and that the sex variable has categories valued from 1 to 2 (_1-2). It then tells you on the right that the category with the value 1 is the omitted (or reference) category. By default, the dummy-variable set is identified by dropping the dummy corresponding to the smallest value of the variable.

So in this case the indicator variable created by Stata is for females (as females are *sex*=2) compared to males. The negative coefficient for the variable _Isex_2 shows the mean difference for women compared to men in logged income. In other words, women on average earn less than men after controlling (adjusting) for age. We can also see from the output that the R^2 value has increased to 0.279 (27.9%) from 6.7% in the model with just *age* and *agesq* as independent variables. This indicates that age and sex explain nearly 28% of the variation in logged income for those in employment.

Next we enter marital status (*mastat*) as an independent variable, also using the **i.** prefix in the following command:

xi:reg ln_inc age agesq i.sex i.mastat

```
. xi:reg ln_inc age agesq i.sex i.mastat
i.sex          _Isex_1-2         (naturally coded; _Isex_1 omitted)
i.mastat       _Imastat_1-6      (naturally coded; _Imastat_1 omitted)

      Source |       SS    df       MS            Number of obs =    4973
-------------+------------------------------      F( 8,  4964) =  255.16
       Model | 686.879702     8 85.8599628        Prob > F      =  0.0000
    Residual | 1670.38419  4964 .336499634        R-squared     =  0.2914
-------------+------------------------------      Adj R-squared =  0.2902
       Total | 2357.26389  4972 .474107781        Root MSE      = .58009


      ln_inc |      Coef.  Std. Err.      t    P>|t|    [95% Conf. Interval]
-------------+----------------------------------------------------------------
         age |   .0939282  .0045723    20.54  0.000    .0849645    .1028919
       agesq |  -.0011177  .0000548   -20.40  0.000   -.0012251   -.0010103
     _Isex_2 |  -.6489609  .0166143   -39.06  0.000   -.6815323   -.6163895
  _Imastat_2 |   .2093674  .0314691     6.65  0.000    .147674     .2710608
  _Imastat_3 |    .310369  .0707913     4.38  0.000    .1715867    .4491513
  _Imastat_4 |   .1887169  .0411138     4.59  0.000    .1081156    .2693181
  _Imastat_5 |   .1691297  .0628323     2.69  0.007    .0459506    .2923088
  _Imastat_6 |   .0238757  .0263734     0.91  0.365   -.0278279    .0755792
       _cons |   5.222049  .0934908    55.86  0.000    5.038766    5.405332
------------------------------------------------------------------------------
```

In this example, the reference category for marital status (*mastat*) is 'married' as that category has the lowest value (1). Remember that the coefficients for the other dummy variables are all compared to the 'married' category. So, for example, category 2 'living as a couple' has a significant coefficient of 0.209 which indicates that those living as a couple, on average, earn more than those who are married, after controlling for age and sex.

If you want your reference categories to be something else, you can change them with the **char** command (short for 'characteristics'). If we wanted to make 'never married' the reference category, then we would use:

char mastat[omit] 6

as the 'never married' category has a value of 6. Now we can rerun the regression command. To restore to the default reference categories type use:

char mastat[omit]

Box 8.2: Using the `xi` command for interactions

The `xi` command also allows us to do interactions easily. The `i.var` syntax is interpreted as follows:

- `i.var1` creates dummies for categorical variable *var1*.
- `i.var1*i.var2` creates dummies for categorical variables *var1* and *var2*: main effects and interactions.
- `i.var1*var3` creates dummies for categorical variable *var1* and includes continuous variable *var3*: all interactions and main effects.
- `i.var1|var3` creates dummies for categorical variable *var1* and includes continuous variable *var3*: all interactions and main effect of *var3*, but not main effect of *var1*.

We can also use the **if** and **bysort** commands with **regress**. For example, if you were interested in running different regression models for each sex then you could use the **if** command:

```
xi:reg ln_inc age agesq i.mastat if sex==1
xi:reg ln_inc age agesq i.mastat if sex==2
```

If you put one or more instances of **i.** in your command you must put the **xi:** first then the **bysort** command:

```
xi: bysort sex: reg ln_inc age agesq i.mastat
```

There are some commands that cannot be combined with **by** and/or **bysort**. If you try to combine them, Stata will give you an error message to this effect.

You could include the indicator or dummy variables by making them using the **tab** command with the **gen** option. For example, using *mastat*=1 as the reference category:

```
tab mastat, gen(mstat)
bysort sex: reg ln_inc age agesq mstat2-mstat6
```

Another slight tweak to the process would be to generate the dummy variables using the **tab** command but then to drop the reference category variable and use an * for all the dummy variables.

Putting an asterisk after the common part of the variable name tells Stata to include all variables that start with that common part; so, **mstat*** will include all variables that start with *mstat*. * is the Stata wildcard notation. So the commands would be:

```
tab mastat, gen(mstat)
drop mstat1
bysort sex: reg ln_inc age agesq mstat*
```

As the **tab** command creates dummy variables for every category of the *mastat* variable, if we did not drop the reference category variable using the * wildcard we would put all dummy variables into the regression. Stata will produce results but it will decide which one of the dummy variables to drop and you lose control over the reference category.

Two of the common options for use with **regress** are:

- **beta**, which requests that normalized beta coefficients be reported instead of confidence intervals;
- **level(#)**, which specifies the confidence level, as a percentage, for confidence intervals of the coefficients.

Regression diagnostics

Stata comes with a series of graphs to help assess whether or not your regression models meet some of the assumptions of linear regression. Using the pull-down menu, these are found at

Graphics → Regression diagnostic plots

Before going on to the diagnostics, we will briefly discuss regression assumptions. Fuller discussions are available in most statistical text books, but we suggest reading Berk (2003) for a general critique of the regression method and its common abuses, while Belsley et al. (2004), Fox (1991) and Pedhazur (1997) are good texts for the assumptions and diagnostics (see also Box 8.3).

The main assumptions of OLS regression are as follows:

1. The independent variables are measured without error.
2. The model is properly specified so that it includes all relevant variables and excludes irrelevant variables.
3. The associations between the independent variables and the dependent variable are linear.

Box 8.3: Errors and ERRORS

One of the things that stuck in our minds as students was a short section in Pedhazur (1997: 9) titled 'There are errors and there are ERRORS', in which he encourages researchers to find the balance between failing to meet the assumptions of statistical techniques (or not caring if they are met or not) and the debilitating quest for statistical perfection in real-world research and data.

Some of the assumptions are testable; others are not and have to be justified by logic and argument. Therefore, no matter how many statistical/diagnostic tests you run there will still be a possibility that you have violated one of the many assumptions. So, to avoid the paralysis of perfection we encourage you to adopt Pedhazur's approach and balance your investigations with some pragmatism: is it an error or an ERROR?

> ... understanding when violations of assumptions lead to serious biases, and when they are of little consequence, are essential to meaningful data analysis.
>
> (Pedhazur 1997: 33).

4. The errors are normally distributed. Errors are the difference between predicted and actual values for each case. Predicted values are also called fitted values. Errors are also called residuals or disturbances.
5. The variance of the errors is constant; usually referred to as homoscedasticity. If the errors do not have constant variance they are heteroscedastic.
6. The errors of one observation are not correlated with the errors of any other observation.
7. The errors are not correlated with any of the independent variables.

Then there are a number of what we call 'technical' issues that you need to check:

8. Strange cases or outliers: these may be from coding errors or may be truly different in which case you may need to examine them further in detail.
9. Leverage and influence: to determine if any of the cases have undue leverage or power on the regression line.

10. Multicollinearity: if the independent variables are highly correlated with one another this may affect the regression estimates.

The first assumption is extremely difficult to meet, if not impossible in social research. Measurement error in the independent variables usually results in underestimating the effects, and the extent of the underestimation has been shown to be linked to the reliability of the measure (Pedhazur 1997). We are guilty of violating this assumption ourselves in the examples in this book. Is the GHQ a completely valid and reliable measure of mental well-being? Not at all, but our models do not take that into account. If you are interested in combining measurement and effect models we suggest you delve into structural equation modelling. It's worth noting that measurement error in the dependent variable does not bias the estimates but does inflate their standard errors, which then gives a higher p value and so a weakened test of significance.

The second assumption, model specification, has to be addressed theoretically, practically, as well as statistically. In developing models to test, the theory needs to be complete, and testable, for the model to be correctly specified. Practical issues such as data availability may also hinder you in specifying a correct model. There are commands in Stata that test whether you have omitted relevant variables. They don't tell you what they are! Nor do they tell you if you have included irrelevant variables. We cover the **linktest** and **ovtest** commands as we go through our example.

The third assumption of linearity is a variation on the second assumption, and we have already discussed ways of dealing with non-linear associations. There are tests for non-linearity but we suggest that these are largely unnecessary if you conduct in-depth univariate and bivariate data analysis before moving on to multivariate analysis.

The distribution of the errors/residuals can be easily attended to after a regression command and the distribution can be visually inspected in graphs and then formally tested using the normality tests covered in Chapter 5. We look at the **rdplot** and **qnorm** graphs as well as summary statistics commands such as **su** and **tabstat** combined with appropriate normality tests in our example.

To see if the variance of the errors is homoscedastic we can plot the errors (residuals) against the predicted (fitted) values in a scatterplot. In such a plot we are looking for no discernable pattern and that the residuals are in an even band across all of the predicted values. This is created by the **rvfplot** command. We can formally test this using the **hettest** command.

The sixth assumption of non-correlated errors is difficult to assess, and with most non-experimental data it is probably safer to assume that these exist, rather than that they don't! Cluster sampling strategies will almost certainly mean this assumption is violated. Again, we have fallen foul of this assumption in our examples as we are using household data and the people who share the same household are probably more alike than those who don't. The effect is to underestimate the standard errors of the coefficients of the independent variables, possibly giving coefficients statistical significance when they shouldn't. A common solution when using cross-sectional data is to use robust standard errors. This can be done in our regression by either using **vce(robust)** as an option or, better, as we know that individuals are clustered in households in our data, the **cluster(hid)** option:

```
xi:reg ln_inc age agesq i.sex i.mastat, ///
     cluster(hid)
```

See what happens to the standard errors, t values and p values compared to the original, partial, output shown below. The coefficients have remained the same but the standard errors have increased resulting in lower t values:

```
    age |   .0939282 .0050763   18.50 0.000   .0839764     .10388
  agesq |  -.0011177 .0000608  -18.39 0.000  -.0012369  -.0009985
 _Isex_2 |  -.6489609 .0166627  -38.95 0.000  -.6816271  -.6162947

    age |   .0939282 .0045723   20.54 0.000   .0849645    .1028919
  agesq |  -.0011177 .0000548  -20.40 0.000  -.0012251  -.0010103
 _Isex_2 |  -.6489609 .0166143  -39.06 0.000  -.6815323  -.6163895
```

The last assumption is linked to model specification, especially in non-experimental data. It follows that if there is an omitted variable that is also correlated with one of the independent variables then, as the effect of that omitted variable is in the error term, then the errors will be correlated with the independent variable. For example, suppose we were investigating children's educational attainment with a model that had parents' education, social class, residence area and number of siblings as independent variables. Parents' income is not available and so is not in the model. However, we know that parents' education and income are likely to be correlated. Therefore, the error term, which includes the effect of parents' income, will be correlated with the included independent variable parents' education.

The three technical issues are discussed more as we work through our example.

We suggest that you adopt a systematic approach to regression diagnostics, and as the diagnostic commands to be used after every regression are generic you could easily copy and paste a set of diagnostic commands into a do file after each regression. This way you know that you haven't missed anything. Such an annotated do file is shown in Box 8.4.

Box 8.4: Diagnostic commands

This summary of Stata commands and the assumption or technical issue they help check for is adapted from Chen et al. (2003).

Model specification
`linktest`	performs a link test for model specification.
`ovtest`	performs regression specification error test for omitted variables.

Normality of errors
`rdplot`	graphs a histogram of the residuals. Use `findit rdplot` to install.
`pnorm`	graphs a standardized normal probability plot.
`swilk`	performs the Shapiro–Wilk *W*-test for normality.

Homoscedasticity
`rvfplot`	graphs residual-versus-fitted plot.
`hettest`	performs Cook and Weisberg test for heteroscedasticity.

Leverage and influence
`predict`	create predicted values, residuals, and measures of influence.
`rvfplot`	graphs residual-versus-fitted plot.
`lvr2plot`	graphs a leverage-versus-squared-residual plot.
`dfbeta`	calculates DFBETAs for all the independent variables.

Multicollinearity
   vif   calculates the variance inflation factor for the independent variables.

An example do file for regression diagnostics is shown below. There are other tests and graphs that you may wish to add later.

```
** Model Specification **
linktest  /* performs a link test
          for model specification
          Look for _hat being sig p<.05
          and _hatsq being not sig p>.05
          _hatsq not sig means no
          omitted vars if _hatsq sig
          then omitted vars */

ovtest    /* performs regression
          specification error test
          for omitted variables. Look
          for p>.05 so not to reject
          hypothesis: model has no
          omitted vars*/

** Normality of errors **
predict res,res        /* use predict to
                       create new var res
                       (residuals) */
predict stres, rsta    /* use predict to
                       create standardized
                       res */

rdplot  /* graphs a histogram of the
        residuals
        Look for a normal distribution
        with no outliers */
** save graph?

** if you haven't installed rdplot then use:
histogram res

pnorm res  /* graphs a standardized normal
           probability (P-P) plot of res
```

```
            Look for plot to be close to
            diagonal */
** save graph?

su res stres  /* summary statistics for
              res
              Look for mean=0 and no min
              and max values >abs 2.5 */
swilk res     /* performs the Shapiro-Wilk
              W test for normality on
              res testing hypothesis of
              normality so p<.05
              rejects */

sktest res    /* for larger samples
              testing hypothesis of
              normality so p<.05
              rejects */

tabstat res, s(sk kur)  /* to actually see
                        the skew and kurt
                        stats remember no
                        skew = 0, no
                        kurt = 3 */

** Homoscedasticity **
rvfplot /* graphs residual-versus-fitted
        plot
        Look for even distribution "no
        pattern" and possible cases of
        high influence */
** save graph?

hettest /* performs Cook and Weisberg
        test for heteroscedasticity
        testing hypothesis of constant
        variance so p<.05 rejects */

** Leverage and influence **
predict lev, leverage  /* create leverage
                       values critical
                       value 2(k+1)/N */
```

```
predict cooks, cooksd   /* create Cook's
                        D stats critical
                        value 4/N */

dfbeta                  /* calculates
                        DFBETAs for all
                        the independent
                        variables critical
                        value 2/sqroot N */

su lev cooks DF*        /* summary stats
                        for inspection and
                        checking against
                        critical values */

lvr2plot   /* graphs a leverage-versus-
           squared-residual plot
           Look for cases with large
           leverage values */

** Multicollinearity **
vif  /* calculates the variance inflation
     factor for ind vars
     Look for VIF > 10 or 1/VIF
     (tolerance) < 0.1 */

drop res stres lev cooks DF*   /*otherwise
                               error
                               after next
                               regession! */
```

A feature of the estimation procedures in Stata is the post-estimation commands; type **help postest** for an introduction. However, there is usually more specific information about post-estimation commands in the sections on the estimation commands, such as **regress**, themselves. Many of the post-estimation commands we cover here are straightforward to apply after a **regress** command, but the results can be obtained in other ways (no surprise there, then!) and most is done through the **predict** command and its options.

We now follow on from our regression example where we had income with a logarithmic transformation as the dependent variable and then age, age squared, sex, and marital status as independent variables in a sample of employed people. While these independent variables explain almost 30% of the variance in logged income, we are not expecting this to be a satisfactory model as we all could think of a number of other factors that would have an effect on income. However, let's proceed with the diagnostics for that model using the do file commands in Box 8.4

First, we use the two tests of model specification: **linktest** and **ovtest**. These tests use a similar process whereby new variables are created and then tested in the model. The **linktest** results are more transparent as they are displayed as a usual regression output, whereas the **ovtest** produces just a single test statistic and its *p* value. We have annotated the do file to indicate what to look for in these test results so you can see that both indicate that we have omitted variables, which is not a surprise.

```
. ** Model Specification **
. linktest  /* performs a link test for model specification
>           Look for _hat being sig p<.05 and _hatsq being not
>           sig p>.05
>           _hatsq not sig means no omitted vars
>           if _hatsq sig then omitted vars */
```

Source	SS	df	MS		
Model	691.771172	2	345.885586		
Residual	1665.49272	4970	.335109198		
Total	2357.26389	4972	.474107781		

Number of obs = 4973
F(2, 4970) = 1032.16
Prob > F = 0.0000
R-squared = 0.2935
Adj R-squared = 0.2932
Root MSE = .57889

ln_inc	Coef.	Std. Err.	t	P>|t|	[95% Conf. Interval]
_hat	-2.007193	.7874233	-2.55	0.011	-3.550891 -.4634963
_hatsq	.2246087	.0587899	3.82	0.000	.1093546 .3398627
_cons	10.03438	2.630634	3.81	0.000	4.877174 15.19158

```
.
. ovtest  /* performs regression specification error test for
>                    omitted variables
>          Look for p>.05 so not to reject hypothesis: model
>                    has no omitted vars*/
Ramsey RESET test using powers of the fitted values of ln_inc
       Ho: model has no omitted variables
             F(3, 4961) = 44.95
             Prob > F   = 0.0000
```

In this next step we use the **predict** command to create two new variables: one for the errors or residuals and one for the standardized residuals. We examine the distribution of the errors

Box 8.5: Alternative diagnostic commands

The `linktest` command can be replicated by:

```
predict yhat, xb
gen yhatsq=yhat^2
reg ln_inc yhat yhatsq
```

The `xb` option to `predict` creates a new variable of the predicted (fitted) values of Y for each case.

The `rdplot` can also be produced by:

```
predict res, r
histogram res
```

The `r` option to `predict` creates a new variable of the residuals (error) for each case. You may also want to examine standardized residuals, in which case use the `rsta` option and graph these.

```
predict stres, rsta
histogram stres
```

The `rvfplot` can also be produced (assuming you have already created the *yhat* and *res* variables) by:

```
scatter res yhat
```

r residuals by first visually inspecting two graphs. The **rdplot** command needs to be installed, so type **findit rdplot** and follow the instructions (see also Box 8.5). If you haven't done this, you can still use **histogram res** to get a similar graph. The histogram shows that there is a longer negative tail on the distribution, indicating that it is probably negatively skewed. In the **norm** graph there is also a departure from the diagonal. You may also want to add a **qnorm** plot here.

```
predict res,res      /* use predict to create
                        new var res (residuals) */
predict stres, rsta  /* use predict to create
                        standardized res */
```

```
.  ** Normality of errors **
.  rdplot   /* graphs a histogram of the residuals
>            Look for a normal distribution
>            with no outliers */
```

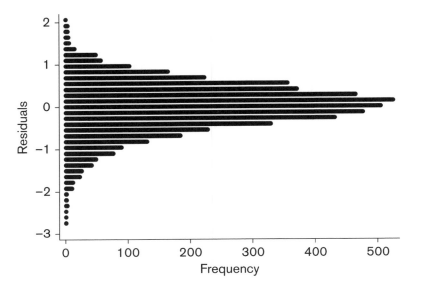

```
.  pnorm res   /* graphs a standardized normal
>              probability (P-P) plot of res
>              Look for plot to be close to
>              diagonal */
```

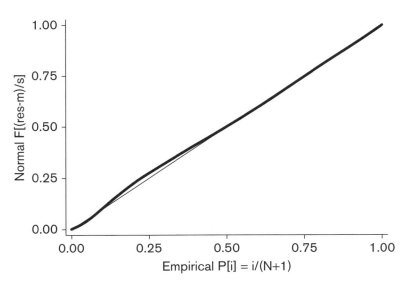

Next, we inspect the summary statistics of the two new variables of the residuals and the standardized residuals using the **su** command. We can see that there are cases with standardized residuals considerably larger than 3, or even 3.5. This indicates that we probably have outliers and that the residuals may not be normally distributed.

```
. su res stres   /* summary statistics for res
                    Look for mean=0 and no min and max
                    values >abs 2.5 */

. su res stres

Variable |   Obs       Mean  Std. Dev.       Min        Max
---------+--------------------------------------------------
     res | 4973  -1.47e-10   .579619  -2.696645   2.102549
   stres | 4973  -.0000186  1.000119  -4.660335   3.403345
```

We formally test the distribution of the errors using the normality tests shown in Chapter 5. These also confirm that the distribution departs from normality in both skewness and kurtosis.

```
. swilk res  /* performs the Shapiro-Wilk W test for
>               normality on res testing hypothesis of
>               normality so p<.05 rejects */

             Shapiro-Wilk W test for normal data
Variable |     Obs         W         V         z     Prob>z
---------+--------------------------------------------------
     res |    4973   0.98902    29.619     8.889    0.00000
```

```
.
. sktest res /* for larger samples
>               testing hypothesis of normality so p<.05
                rejects */

             Skewness/Kurtosis tests for Normality
                                    ------ joint ------
Variable | Pr(Skewness) Pr(Kurtosis) adj chi2(2) Prob>chi2
---------+--------------------------------------------------
     res |       0.000        0.000          .      0.0000
```

```
.
. tabstat res, s(sk kur) /* to actually see the skew and
>         kurt stats remember no skew = 0, no kurt = 3 */

variable |    skewness    kurtosis
---------+----------------------------
     res |   -.4042151     3.79337
------------------------------------
```

The visual inspection of the graph of fitted values (predicted values) against residuals (errors) clearly shows that the variance of the errors is not constant across the range of fitted values. Therefore, we have violated the assumption of homoscedasticity. This is confirmed by the statistical test which rejects the hypothesis of constant variance.

```
. ** Homoscedasticity **
. rvfplot  /* graphs residual-versus-fitted plot
>            Look for even distribution "no
>            pattern" and possible cases of high
>            influence */
```

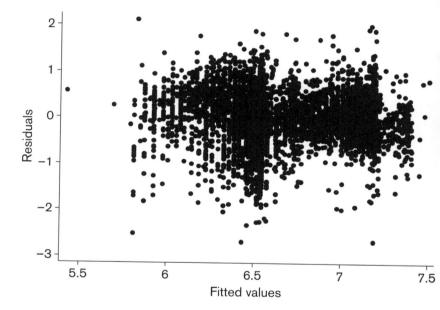

```
. hettest  /* performs Cook and Weisberg test
>            for heteroscedasticity testing
>            hypothesis of constant variance so
>            p<.05 rejects */

Breusch-Pagan / Cook-Weisberg test for
heteroskedasticity
         Ho: Constant variance
         Variables: fitted values of ln_inc

         chi2(1)     = 190.58
         Prob > chi2 = 0.0000
```

For this next part of the diagnostics we create the leverage and influence values for each case in new variables. The leverage and Cook's D values are created using the **predict** command, and the **dfbeta** command automatically produces a DFBETA value for all the independent variables. We then use the **su** command to make a table so that we can see if any of the values are greater than the critical values. This isn't the place to engage in a debate on the use of critical values or cut-offs, but just to say that these are *rules of thumb* rather than commandments set in stone. One point to think about is the effect of having N in the denominator in these calculations when using samples in the many thousands. In our current model we have eight independent variables so $k = 8$, and an estimation sample of 4973 so $N = 4973$. Accordingly, the critical values are: leverage, 0.00362; Cook's D, 0.0008; and DFBETA, 0.02836. All of the values indicate that there are cases that have undue leverage and/or influence in this model. The leverage–residual plot clearly shows that there are quite a few cases with high leverage values.

```
** Leverage and influence **
predict lev, leverage  /* create leverage values
                             critical value 2(k+1)/N */
predict cooks, cooksd  /* create Cook's D stats
                             critical value 4/N */
dfbeta                 /* calculates DFBETAs for all the
                             independent variables
                             critical value 2/sqroot N */
              DFage:  DFbeta(age)
            DFagesq:  DFbeta(agesq)
          DF_Isex_2:  DFbeta(_Isex_2)
       DF_Imastat_2:  DFbeta(_Imastat_2)
       DF_Imastat_3:  DFbeta(_Imastat_3)
       DF_Imastat_4:  DFbeta(_Imastat_4)
       DF_Imastat_5:  DFbeta(_Imastat_5)
       DF_Imastat_6:  DFbeta(_Imastat_6)

su lev cooks DF*  /* summary stats for inspection and
                     checking against critical values */
```

Variable	Obs	Mean	Std. Dev.	Min	Max
lev	4973	.0018098	.0024166	.0006241	.0229986
cooks	4973	.0001882	.0005523	1.84e-14	.0227647
F_Imastat_2	4973	-2.97e-07	.0128734	-.1459199	.1329711
F_Imastat_3	4973	-3.84e-07	.0125399	-.2566079	.1986158
F_Imastat_4	4973	-3.33e-07	.0129498	-.2335146	.1920423
F_Imastat_5	4973	2.39e-08	.0123927	-.197925	.2329337
F_Imastat_6	4973	-1.03e-06	.0135859	-.1608311	.1074181
DFage	4973	-2.23e-06	.0158038	-.3712751	.1422175
DFagesq	4973	2.53e-06	.0158053	-.1336512	.4085968
DF_Isex_2	4973	2.31e-06	.0142373	-.0704291	.0673829

```
lvr2plot  /* graphs a leverage-versus-squared-residual plot
             Look for cases with large leverage values */
```

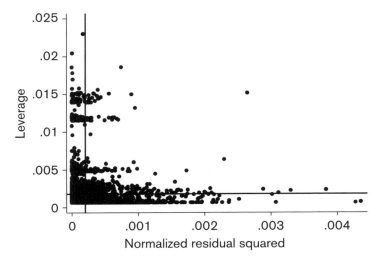

Finally, we examine whether any of the independent variable are collinear as a check for multicollinearity. As a precursor to regression you should be looking at the bivariate association between potential independent variables which would give an early warning about issues of multicollinearity. The **vif** command produces the variance inflation factor and the tolerance which is simply the reciprocal of the variance inflation factor and preferred by some users. Our results show that there is collinearity between age and age squared, but is to be expected as they have an almost perfect linear correlation! All of the other independent variables have variance inflation factors less than 10 or tolerance greater than 0.1, which shows that multicollinearity does not exist.

```
. ** Multicollinearity **
. vif  /* calculates the variance inflation factor for ind var
>      Look for VIF > 10 or 1/VIF (tolerance) < 0.1 */

    Variable |      VIF     1/VIF
-------------+----------------------
         age |    46.83   0.021356
       agesq |    43.17   0.023162
  _Imastat_6 |     1.70   0.586526
  _Imastat_2 |     1.16   0.861387
  _Imastat_3 |     1.06   0.946293
  _Imastat_4 |     1.03   0.972071
     _Isex_2 |     1.02   0.980591
  _Imastat_5 |     1.01   0.986029
-------------+----------------------
    Mean VIF |    12.12

.
. drop res stres lev cooks DF*   /*otherwise error after next
                                   regession! */
```

So, what does all this mean for our regression model? In terms of model specification, it is not surprising that these results indicate that we have omitted variables; no one would think that age, sex and marital status alone would satisfactorily explain variations in income. Some of the omitted variables could be education, work experience, and sector of industry, for example. The errors or residuals are well dispersed beyond the normal distribution, with some standardized residuals beyond 3.5. The error terms are also heteroscedastic, which is more than likely linked with the poor model specification. A good number of cases have large leverage and/or influence which could be linked to the outliers seen in the residuals, but not necessarily so. However, we are confident that we do not have multicollinearity, which is at least one thing going for this model at this stage. Clearly, quite a lot more work needs to be done before we obtain a more satisfactory model.

LOGISTIC REGRESSION

Logistic regression (also called logit or, to distinguish it from other types of categorical dependent variables, binary logit or binary logistic regression) is used for regression with a dichotomous dependent variable. Stata's **logit** command has the same general format as **regress**. The dependent variable should be a 0/1 dichotomy; for analytic purposes a 0 is referred to as a failure and 1 as a success, regardless of the substantive meaning of the variables. For more discussion on the details and application of logistic regression, see Long (1997), Long and Freese (2006), or Menard (2002).

Many users prefer the **logistic** command to **logit**. Results are the same regardless of which you use, but the **logistic** command reports odds ratios (Box 8.6) rather than logit coefficients by default.

In this example, we will look at the outcome of whether or not a person has a first degree or higher, derived from the variable *educ* (for the variable *educ*, higher degree = 1, first degree = 2). Therefore, to construct the dichotomous or binary variable:

```
recode educ (1/2=1) (3/max=0),gen(degree)
```

We will also use the whole sample of the example data. So, if we were following on from the above example looking at income as

the dependent variable in a sample of those working, we woul
need to open the data again. And not forgetting to recode th
missing values as well!

As the sample contains people aged 16 and older, it is unlikel
that the younger people in the sample would have had the oppo
tunity to gain a degree so we'll restrict this analysis to those age
25 and older by using the command

drop if age<25

First, we will examine if sex and age are determinants of hav
ing a degree:

xi:logit degree i.sex age

```
. xi:logit degree i.sex age
i.sex          _Isex_1-2          (naturally coded; _Isex_1 omitted

Iteration 0:  log likelihood = -2301.563
Iteration 1:  log likelihood = -2189.489
Iteration 2:  log likelihood = -2180.6155
Iteration 3:  log likelihood = -2180.5053
Iteration 4:  log likelihood = -2180.5053

Logistic regression                      Number of obs =     839
                                         LR chi2(2)    =  242.1
                                         Prob > chi2   = 0.000
Log likelihood = -2180.5053              Pseudo R2     = 0.052

-----------------------------------------------------------------
 degree |    Coef. Std. Err.      z  P>|z|  [95% Conf. Interval
--------+--------------------------------------------------------
_Isex_2 | -.4637623  .0830406  -5.58 0.000  -.6265189 -.301005
    age | -.0406401  .0030834 -13.18 0.000  -.0466835 -.034596
  _cons |  -.423095  .1381117  -3.06 0.002   -.693789 -.15240
-----------------------------------------------------------------
```

Compare the output from the **logit** command above with th
output from the **logistic** command below. You can see tha
odds ratios are presented instead of coefficients but the z and
values are identical, as are the model fit statistics reported in th
top right-hand panel.

xi:logistic degree i.sex age

```
 xi:logistic degree i.sex age
.sex          _Isex_1-2              (naturally coded; _Isex_1 omitted)
ogistic regression                           Number of obs = 8390
                                             LR chi2(2)    = 242.12
                                             Prob > chi2   = 0.0000
og likelihood = -2180.5053                   Pseudo R2     = 0.0526
-------------------------------------------------------------------
degree | Odds Ratio Std. Err.      z P>|z|  [95% Conf. Interval]
-------+-----------------------------------------------------------
Isex_2 |    .628913  .0522253   -5.58 0.000   .5344491   .7400735
   age |   .9601746  .0029606  -13.18 0.000   .9543894   .9659949
-------------------------------------------------------------------
```

Jsing the **or** option with the **logit** command will give you the
ame results as using the **logistic** command, such as:

ogit degree i.sex age, or

Box 8.6: Odds ratios

Odds ratios are sometimes preferred over logit coefficients for
their ease of interpretation. The logit coefficients report the effect
of the independent variable on the logarithm of the odds of being
in the 1 category of the dependent variable compared to being in
the 0 category. Or, in our example, of having a degree compared to
not having one. So, the logit coefficient for *sex* in our example is
−0.464 which we would interpret as saying that women have, on
average, 0.464 less of the logarithm of the odds of having a degree.

Odds ratios are the exponential of the logit coefficient. Here
we simply take the exponential of the logit coefficient using the
calculator in Stata:

display exp(-.464)

```
. display exp(-.464)
.62876355
```

So, the odds ratio for the variable *sex* is 0.63. Odds ratios range
from 0 to +∞, with the value for no effect being equal to 1. This
means that odds ratios lower than 1 are 'negative' effects and odds
ratios greater than 1 are 'positive' effects. The odds ratio of 0.63 in
our example is interpreted as 37% less likely to have a degree. An
odds ratio of 1.43 would be interpreted as 43% more likely, and
so on. As you may gather, the range above 1 is greater than that
below 1, which is bounded by zero, so comparing the magnitude
of effects either side of 1 is not straightforward and needs care.

Even though these results indicate that women are less likely t have a degree than men (odds ratio 0.63) and that as age increase the likelihood is reduced (odds ratio 0.96), it is unlikely that th gender difference is constant with all values of age, as we know that in the past much fewer women went to university. It is there fore possible that there is an interaction between age and sex i that the effect of age varies across sexes. For more details on inte action effects in logistic regression, see Jaccard (2001). We can te this by including an interaction term as described in Box 8.2:

xi: logistic degree i.sex*age

```
. xi:logistic degree i.sex*age
i.sex           _Isex_1-2         (naturally coded; _Isex_1 omitted
i.sex*age       _IsexXage_#       (coded as above)

Logistic regression                        Number of obs  = 8390
                                           LR chi2(3)     = 250.6
                                           Prob > chi2    = 0.000
Log likelihood = -2176.2561                Pseudo R2      = 0.054

------------------------------------------------------------------
     degree | Odds Ratio Std. Err.      z P>|z|  [95% Conf. Interval]
------------+-----------------------------------------------------
    _Isex_2 |   1.324136   .356577   1.04 0.297   .7811104   2.24467
        age |   .9677965  .0038777  -8.17 0.000   .9602261   .97542
_IsexXage_2 |   .9819062  .0062061  -2.89 0.004   .9698176   .99414
------------------------------------------------------------------
```

The results indicate that the interaction term (_IsexXage_2) ha a significant coefficient which tells us that the effect of age vari across sexes or, conversely, the effect of sex varies with age.

To get a clearer picture of what this means it's a good id to graph interaction effects. We can easily do this by using th **predict** post-estimation command to calculate predicted, fitted, values.

predict yhat,xb

Then use the pull-down menu:

Graphics → Twoway graph

Then create two plots in a similar way to that described Box 6.7 but with the following entries:

lot1: **X axis** = *age*, **Y axis** = *yhat*, **if/in** tab – sex==1
lot 2: **X axis** = *age*, **Y axis** = *yhat*, **if/in** tab – sex==2
egend tab – select **Override default keys** and type 1 'men'
    2 'women' in the box.

dd titles as you wish.

The graph shows that with increasing age both men and
omen are less likely to have a degree than younger people. But
hen looking at the effect of age on each sex, you can see that at
ge 25 there is little difference in the likelihood of having a degree
ut that the gap increases as age increases. Therefore, the gender
ap increases as age increases, which makes substantive sense
om what we know about recent history of university admissions
nd accessibility. It is worth noting that the Y-axis units are in
git (log of the odds). Compare this with the results shown in
ox 8.7.

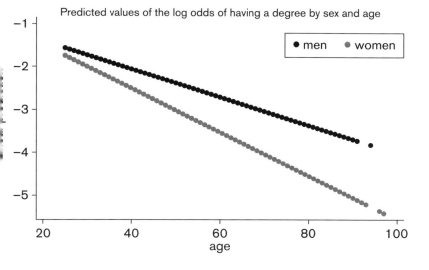

Predicted values of the log odds of having a degree by sex and age

THER REGRESSION COMMANDS

asic regression commands in Stata generally have the same struc-
ıre in that the command is followed by the dependent variable
nd then a list of independent variables. There are many other
gression models; if you wish to extend your knowledge of
gression models with categorical or count dependent variables,
ıen we recommend you use Long (1997) or Long and Freese
!006).

Box 8.7: Post-estimation commands

There are a series of very useful post-estimation commands available to download if your copy of Stata is web enabled. These are based on the **spostado** commands developed by Long and Freese (2006). You must first install the **spostado** files which can be found by typing **findit spostado**. The new box will show a link to:

spost9_ado from http://www.indiana.edu/ ~jslsoc/stata

Click on this link which will take you to another new box and then simply click where it says **click here to install**.

Follow the same three steps to install the **postgr3** and **xi3** commands developed by Michael Mitchell and Phil Ender at UCLA: Academic Technology Services, Statistical Consulting Group. See www.ats.ucla.edu/stat/stata/ado/analysis/.

Now rerun the logistic regression using the **xi3** prefix:

xi3: logistic degree i.sex*age

```
. xi3:logistic degree i.sex*age
i.sex     _Isex_1-2     (naturally coded; _Isex_1 omitted)

Logistic regression                        Number of obs =     8390
                                           LR chi2(3)    =   250.61
                                           Prob > chi2   =   0.0000
Log likelihood = -2176.2561                Pseudo R2     =   0.0544

---------------------------------------------------------------------
  degree | Odds Ratio Std. Err.     z  P>|z|  [95% Conf. Interval]
---------+-----------------------------------------------------------
 _Isex_2 |   1.324136   .356577  1.04  0.297    .7811104   2.244672
     age |   .9677965  .0038777 -8.17  0.000    .9602261   .9754266
_Ise2Xag |   .9819062  .0062061 -2.89  0.004    .9698176   .9941455
---------------------------------------------------------------------
```

Then use the **postgr3** command to produce a graph of the probability of having a degree by age for both men and women. The lines for men and women are produced by using the **by(sex)** option. Try omitting this and see what graph is produced. The graph varies from the one produced by using linear fitted values as this one has probability of having a degree on the Y axis. In some ways this is easier to understand than fitted logit values. There are many other ways to use this, and other post-estimation graphing commands. For more information, see Long and Freese (2006) and the UCLA website.

```
. postgr3 age,by(sex)
Variables left asis: age _Isex_2 _Ise2Xag
```

Here in brief are some of the more common regression commands:

mlogit – multinomial logit regression for nominal dependent variables with three or more categories. Note that there is *not* a mlogistic command. Relative risk ratios are reported if the **rrr** option is used.
ologit – ordered logit regression for an ordinal dependent variable. Again, there is *not* an ologistic command, but if you wish to show odds ratios then use the **or** option.
probit – binary probit regression. Probit is the other main method for analysing binary dependent variables. Whereas logit (or logistic) regression is based on log odds, probit uses the cumulative normal probability distribution.
mprobit – multinomial probit regression. Probit for nominal dependent variables with three or more categories.
oprobit – ordered probit regression. Probit for an ordinal dependent variable.
poisson – Poisson regression for a count (non-negative integers) dependent variable.

- **nbreg** – negative binomial regression for a count variable that is overdispersed. A Poisson distribution is a special case of the negative binomial family, and a dependent variable with a true Poisson distribution can also be estimated using the **nbreg** command.

Box 8.8: Weighting

If your data is simply weighted then Stata can use the weights in a number of ways, depending on how and why the weights were constructed – see **help weight**. Weighting is a complicated (and controversial) issue and it is beyond the scope of this book to go into the whys and wherefores of it. Briefly, you can weight tables and most estimation procedures by adding a weight option to the command line in square brackets. Here we show two examples of using weights in a crosstabulation and in a regression model. The weighting variable is *weight*.

```
ta mastat sex [aw=weight]
xi:reg ghqscale i.sex age i.mastat [pw=weight]
```

Box 8.9: Applications of regression modelling in a research project

In a series of analyses using data from the first wave of the Canadian National Longitudinal Survey of Children and Youth (NLSCY) we were interested in the factors associated with birth outcomes (low birthweight, preterm birth and small for gestational age) and then how birth outcomes affected motor and social development in very young children.

In the first analysis[1] we had three dichotomous birthweight outcomes. Low birthweight (LBW) was defined as those children born weighing less than 2500 g, preterm birth was birth at 258 days' gestation or less, and small for gestational age (SGA) was defined as those under the 10th percentile of the gestational growth curves. These dichotomous outcomes were the dependent variables in a series of logistic regression models with social, environmental and mother's behavioural variables as independent variables. We presented our results as odds ratios as we categorized all of our independent variables and used dummy variables so they could show either an increased or decreased risk of either LBW or SGA compared to the reference category of the independent variable.

In the second analysis[2] we examined how birthweight, this time classified as LBW (less than 2500 g) and VLBW (less than 1500 g) compared to normal, was associated with motor and social development at ages up to 48 months net of the effects of family and social variables. The motor and social development (MSD) scale used in the analysis was an interval level scale created from a number of items (see our comments in Box 5.1) which was reasonably normally distributed as the scale creation was designed so that the 'average' child for their age scored 100. This enabled us to use a series of OLS regression models to estimate the effects of the independent variables on the MSD scale. We used nested models to test for mediating effects and also tested for interactions (or moderating effects; see this chapter and Chapter 9). We found that there was a significant interaction between mother's education and birthweight which indicated that the low birthweight children with higher educated mothers had 'normal' MSD scores of about 100, while low birthweight children with mothers with lower education had MSD scores less than 90. We presented this interaction as a graph to better convey the moderating effects of birthweight and education on the MSD scale.

[1] Pevalin, D.J., Wade, T.J., Brannigan, A. and Sauve R. (2001) Beyond biology: The social context of prenatal behaviour and birth outcomes. *Social and Preventive Medicine*, 46: 233–239.

[2] Pevalin, D.J., Wade, T.J. and Brannigan, A. (2003) Parental assessment of early childhood development: Biological and social covariates. *Infant and Child Development*, 12: 167–175.

DEMONSTRATION EXERCISE

In Chapter 3 we manipulated the individual level variables and saved a new data set called demodata1.dta. In Chapter 4 we merged a household level variable indicating the region of the country onto the individual level data and saved the data with a new name demodata2.dta. In Chapter 5 we examined the variables we are using for their distribution, measures of central tendency and, for continuous variables, their normality. In Chapter 6 we examined differences in mean GHQ scale scores across groups in the

factors but did not formally test for differences. The dichotomou
indicator was tested using the **tab** command and measures o
association. Correlations between the GHQ scale and interva
level factors were produced. In Chapter 7 we formally teste
for differences of mean GHQ scores and proportions above th
threshold of the dichotomous GHQ indicator between groups.

At this stage of this demonstration we use multivariate OL
regression with the GHQ scale as the dependent variable and then
use multivariate binary logistic regression with the dichotomou
GHQ indicator as the dependent variable. In these models we us
all of the factors we are interested in to assess their net effects o
mental well-being.

In this first regression model we use the **xi:** prefix as we hav
a number of categorical independent variables which need to b
converted into indicator or dummy variables. We also use the ag
categories to see if the association with age is linear or non-linea

```
xi:reg ghqscale female i.agecat i.marst2 ///
    i.empstat i.numchd i.region2
```

In the output below we have put the significant coefficients in bol
for easier identification. These results indicate that women hav
on average higher GHQ scores by 1.05 points. The second ag
category (33–50 years) has significantly higher GHQ scores than
the reference (youngest) category (18–32 years), whereas the thir
category (51–65 years) is not significantly different from the refer
ence category. This suggests that the association is non-linea
and possibly could be better defined with a quadratic term fo
age. The dummy variables for marital status categories show tha
those who are married are not significantly different from th
reference category (single) but those who are separated or divorce
(category 3) and widowed (category 4) have significantly highe
GHQ scores than those who are single. Most of the people in thi
sample are married, so it may be more appropriate to use the mar
ried category as the reference, and we will change this in the nex
regression model. For employment status, three of the categorie
(unemployed, long term sick and family care) have significantl
higher GHQ scores than the reference category (employed). Thos
with one or two children in the household have significantl
higher GHQ scores than those with no children, but those wit
three or more children are not significantly different from thos
with no children.

```
xi:reg ghqscale female i.agecat i.marst2 i.empstat ///
  i.numchd i.region2
.agecat      _Iagecat_1-3     (naturally coded; _Iagecat_1 omitted)
.marst2      _Imarst2_1-4     (naturally coded; _Imarst2_1 omitted)
.empstat     _Iempstat_1-6    (naturally coded; _Iempstat_1 omitted)
.numchd      _Inumchd_1-3     (naturally coded; _Inumchd_1 omitted)
.region2     _Iregion2_1-7    (naturally coded; _Iregion2_1 omitted)

    Source |       SS       df       MS              Number of obs =    7688
-----------+------------------------------           F( 19,  7668) =   35.04
     Model | 15242.5628      19  802.240149          Prob > F      =  0.0000
  Residual | 175575.003    7668  22.8971053          R-squared     =  0.0799
-----------+------------------------------           Adj R-squared =  0.0776
     Total | 190817.566    7687  24.8234117          Root MSE      =  4.7851


-----------------------------------------------------------------------------
  ghqscale |      Coef.  Std. Err.      t    P>|t|    [95% Conf. Interval]
-----------+-----------------------------------------------------------------
    female |  1.051762   .1179439    8.92   0.000     .8205601    1.282965
_Iagecat_2 |  .3340761   .1366896    2.44   0.015     .0661272     .602025
_Iagecat_3 |  -.075252   .1838687   -0.41   0.682     -.435685     .285181
_Imarst2_2 |  .1601081   .1709917    0.94   0.349    -.1750823    .4952986
_Imarst2_3 |  1.597959   .2581717    6.19   0.000     1.091871    2.104046
_Imarst2_4 |  1.489015   .4102427    3.63   0.000     .6848276    2.293203
_Iempstat_2 | 2.912573   .2282301   12.76   0.000     2.465179    3.359966
_Iempstat_3 | 5.155082   .3274935   15.74   0.000     4.513105    5.797058
_Iempstat_4 |  .5919008   .3422444    1.73   0.084    -.0789917    1.262793
_Iempstat_5 | 1.123951   .1904472    5.90   0.000     .7506226     1.49728
_Iempstat_6 | -.2368232  .2823437   -0.84   0.402     -.790294    .3166477
_Inumchd_2 |  .4985591   .1438261    3.47   0.001     .2166205    .7804976
_Inumchd_3 |  .4114755   .2415769    1.70   0.089    -.0620813    .8850324
_Iregion2_2 | -.2086025  .1956044   -1.07   0.286    -.5920406    .1748356
_Iregion2_3 |  -.172131    .21373   -0.81   0.421    -.5911002    .2468381
_Iregion2_4 | -.2925766  .2381277   -1.23   0.219    -.7593719    .1742188
_Iregion2_5 |  -.141722   .2164165  -0.65   0.513    -.5659575    .2825135
_Iregion2_6 |  .4176472   .2944849   1.42   0.156    -.1596238    .9949182
_Iregion2_7 | -.2650218  .2430078   -1.09   0.275    -.7413834    .2113399
     _cons |  9.322474   .2124677   43.88   0.000      8.90598    9.738969
-----------------------------------------------------------------------------
```

here are no significant differences for the dummy variables
or region of the country compared to the reference category of
ondon. However, if you examine the coefficients more closely
ou can see that category 6 (Wales) is 0.417 higher than the
eference category and category 4 (Northwest) is 0.292 lower than
he reference category. This difference might be significant, but is
ot tested in this model. We can, however, test this with a post-
stimation command:

est _Iregion2_6= _Iregion2_4

```
. test _Iregion2_6= _Iregion2_4

( 1) - _Iregion2_4 + _Iregion2_6 = 0

       F( 1, 7668) = 5.84
          Prob > F = 0.0157
```

The output above tests for a difference between the two coeffici‐ents and the *p* value of the test is less than 0.05 which suggest that they are different. However, for a variable such as *region2* w might want to see if the regions are significantly different from th overall sample mean rather than choose a reference category.

From our observations above, we need to adjust some of th variables and commands to re-estimate this regression model First, we wish to capture the non-linear nature of the associ‐ation between age and GHQ score by adding a squared age term to the model. Therefore, we need to create a new variable fo the squared value of age.

gen age2=age^2

Next, we want to change the reference category for marital statu to married (category 2).

char marst2 [omit] 2

Finally, we want the coefficients for the region categories to b compared to the overall or grand mean in the sample. To do thi we need to have downloaded the **xi3** command/prefix (see Box 8.7 Dummy variables that indicate differences from the grand mea are usually referred to as effect coding, and this is done b prefixing the regression command with **xi3:** and then prefixin the region variable with **e.** (rather than **i.**). So, the new regres sion looks like this:

**xi3:reg ghqscale female age age2 i.marst2 ///
    i.empstat i.numchd e.region2**

```
. xi3:reg ghqscale female age age2 i.marst2 ///
   i.empstat i.numchd e.region2
i.marst2    _Imarst2_1-4    (naturally coded; _Imarst2_2 omitted)
i.empstat   _Iempstat_1-6   (naturally coded; _Iempstat_1 omitted
i.numchd    _Inumchd_1-3    (naturally coded; _Inumchd_1 omitted)
e.region2   _Iregion2_1-7   (naturally coded; _Iregion2_1 omitted
```

```
    Source |       SS    df         MS        Number of obs =    7688
-----------+------------------------------    F( 19,  7668) =   35.66
     Model | 15491.6833    19  815.351754     Prob > F       = 0.0000
  Residual | 175325.883  7668  22.8646169     R-squared      = 0.0812
-----------+------------------------------    Adj R-squared  = 0.0789
     Total | 190817.566  7687  24.8234117     Root MSE       = 4.7817

--------------------------------------------------------------------------
   ghqscale |     Coef.  Std. Err.     t  P>|t|   [95% Conf. Interval]
-----------+--------------------------------------------------------------
     female |  1.045367  .1179395   8.86  0.000    .814173    1.27656
        age |  .1502465  .0342705   4.38  0.000    .083067   .2174259
       age2 | -.0018732   .000422  -4.44  0.000   -.0027005   -.001046
  _Imarst2_1 | -.0464479  .1816749  -0.26  0.798   -.4025804   .3096846
  _Imarst2_3 |  1.415416  .2165824   6.54  0.000    .990855   1.839977
  _Imarst2_4 |  1.438633  .3810207   3.78  0.000    .6917286  2.185538
 _Iempstat_2 |  2.973164  .2288571  12.99  0.000    2.524541  3.421786
 _Iempstat_3 |  5.182441  .3275309  15.82  0.000    4.540391  5.824491
 _Iempstat_4 |  .7544566  .3465094   2.18  0.029    .0752034   1.43371
 _Iempstat_5 |  1.166145  .1902912   6.13  0.000    .7931224  1.539168
 _Iempstat_6 |  .1311709  .3059574   0.43  0.668   -.4685892   .730931
  _Inumchd_2 |  .4154971  .1458797   2.85  0.004    .129533   .7014611
  _Inumchd_3 |  .2894564  .2449152   1.18  0.237   -.1906445   .7695572
  _Iregion2_2 | -.1058743  .1047368  -1.01  0.312   -.3111871   .0994386
  _Iregion2_3 | -.0641072  .1273939  -0.50  0.615   -.3138341   .1856197
  _Iregion2_4 |  -.196559  .1551697  -1.27  0.205    -.500734   .1076161
  _Iregion2_5 | -.0411748  .1305821  -0.32  0.753   -.2971515   .2148019
  _Iregion2_6 |  .5126046  .2130926   2.41  0.016    .0948849   .9303244
  _Iregion2_7 | -.1743432  .1608996  -1.08  0.279   -.4897504    .141064
       _cons |  6.794737   .665037  10.22  0.000    5.491082   8.098391
--------------------------------------------------------------------------
```

The significant coefficients for both the *age* and *age2* variables indicate that we were correct to model a non-linear association, and the positive coefficient for the *age* variable and the negative coefficient for the *age2* variable show that the association first increases with age and then decreases in an inverted U shape.

The categories of marital status show that those separated or divorced and those widowed have significantly higher GHQ scores than those who are married. If you examine the dummy variables for marital status you can see that now category 2 (_Imarst2_2) is missing and is therefore the reference category.

The dummy variables for employment status were not altered but you can see that the coefficient for category 4 (_Iempstat_4) is now significant, which it wasn't in the first regression model. The coefficient is larger, which may have resulted from the better specification of other variables in the model.

The categories of the *region2* variable now show differences from the grand mean of the sample. Now they indicate that category 6 (_Iregion2_6) has significantly higher GHQ scores than the sample average. You can see that even though the coefficients now show difference from the grand mean, one of the categories is still missing. If you wish to find the difference for this category then you can rerun the regression omitting another category of the region2 variable. Omitting category 2 produces the following extract of results:

```
_Iregion2_1 |    .0694538   .1555509    0.45   0.655   -.2354686    .374376
_Iregion2_3 |   -.0641072   .1273939   -0.50   0.615   -.3138341    .185619
_Iregion2_4 |    -.196559   .1551697   -1.27   0.205    -.500734    .107616
_Iregion2_5 |   -.0411748   .1305821   -0.32   0.753   -.2971515    .214801
_Iregion2_6 |    .5126046   .2130926    2.41   0.016    .0948849    .930324
_Iregion2_7 |   -.1743432   .1608996   -1.08   0.279   -.4897504    .14106
```

Box 8.10: Graphing effect coded categorical variables

Effect coding categorical independent variables gives you the opportunity to graph the information in a way that is intuitively attractive and logical. Copy and paste the regression results into an Excel spreadsheet (see Chapter 2) and then add the coefficient and confidence interval for the omitted category from rerunning the regression with another category omitted (by using the **char** command). Now you can graph the categories' differences from the grand mean along with the 95% confidence interval, and the resulting graph shows very clearly that, on average, Wales has significantly higher GHQ scores than the sample average after controlling for sex, age, marital status, employment status and number of children.

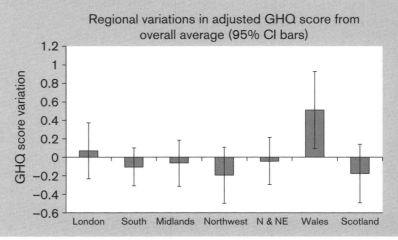

Regional variations in adjusted GHQ score from overall average (95% CI bars)

Alternatively, you can add the coefficient from all the other categories, and then the difference from zero is the omitted coefficient. For example, from the extract, $0.06945 - 0.06410 - 0.19655 - 0.04117 + 0.51260 - 0.17434 = 0.10587$. The difference from zero is -0.10587 (as with effect coding all the differences add to zero, see Box 8.10) which, if you check the previous output, is the coefficient for category 2 (_Iregion2_2).

Now we run a logistic regression using the binary GHQ indicator (d_ghq) and the same independent variables as on p. 312.

```
xi3:logistic d_ghq female i.agecat i.marst2 ///
    i.empstat i.numchd e.region2
```

```
xi3:logistic d_ghq female i.agecat i.marst2 ///
  i.empstat i.numchd e.region2
.agecat     _Iagecat_1-3     (naturally coded; _Iagecat_1 omitted)
.marst2     _Imarst2_1-4     (naturally coded; _Imarst2_2 omitted)
.empstat    _Iempstat_1-6    (naturally coded; _Iempstat_1 omitted)
.numchd     _Inumchd_1-3     (naturally coded; _Inumchd_1 omitted)
.region2    _Iregion2_1-7    (naturally coded; _Iregion2_1 omitted)
```

```
ogistic regression                          Number of obs  =    7688
                                            LR chi2(19)    = 339.92
                                            Prob > chi2    = 0.0000
og likelihood = -3536.4272                  Pseudo R2      = 0.0459
```

d_ghq	Odds Ratio	Std. Err.	z	P>|z|	[95% Conf. Interval]	
female	1.389437	.0920517	4.96	0.000	1.220242	1.582093
_Iagecat_2	.9136479	.0672408	-1.23	0.220	.7909223	1.055417
_Iagecat_3	.7308843	.0755579	-3.03	0.002	.5968326	.8950448
_Imarst2_1	.906441	.0862042	-1.03	0.302	.752296	1.09217
_Imarst2_3	1.733206	.1806035	5.28	0.000	1.413036	2.125921
_Imarst2_4	1.521458	.2964534	2.15	0.031	1.038496	2.229026
_Iempstat_2	3.248623	.3395573	11.27	0.000	2.646847	3.987217
_Iempstat_3	5.355798	.7744645	11.61	0.000	4.034019	7.11067
_Iempstat_4	1.39944	.2578951	1.82	0.068	.975194	2.008249
_Iempstat_5	1.406923	.1355923	3.54	0.000	1.164758	1.699437
_Iempstat_6	.8380977	.1500266	-0.99	0.324	.5900955	1.190329
_Inumchd_2	1.175711	.0914464	2.08	0.037	1.009472	1.369326
_Inumchd_3	1.041569	.1355878	0.31	0.754	.8070155	1.344295
_Iregion2_2	.9657438	.055782	-0.60	0.546	.8623746	1.081503
_Iregion2_3	.9555518	.0665694	-0.65	0.514	.8335937	1.095353
_Iregion2_4	.9810842	.0826423	-0.23	0.821	.8317729	1.157198
_Iregion2_5	.9029198	.0653833	-1.41	0.158	.7834493	1.040609
_Iregion2_6	1.344802	.1439638	2.77	0.006	1.090274	1.658751
_Iregion2_7	.8339696	.076168	-1.99	0.047	.6972819	.997452

The results of the logistic regression show similar associations t
those in the OLS regression models. One noticeable difference i
the association with age. In the OLS models the association wa
non-linear and best captured with a quadratic term, but the abov
output, using dummy variables for the age categories (shaded
shows a decreasing likelihood of being over the GHQ threshol
with age, thus suggesting that a linear term can capture the associa
tion. Using the interval-level *age* variable produced the followin
coefficient in the logistic regression (other output omitted):

```
---------------------------------------------------------------------
   d_ghq | Odds Ratio Std. Err.     z  P>|z|  [95% Conf.Interval]
---------+-----------------------------------------------------------
  female |   1.386245  .0918595  4.93  0.000   1.217405 1.578501
     age |   .9895113  .0030573 -3.41  0.001   .9835373 .9955217
```

9 Presenting your Results

In this chapter, we will take you through some techniques for presenting your results to a scientific or policy audience. This part of research is given far less attention than it should be. It is one thing to produce a bunch of statistical findings – it is quite another to be able to communicate them clearly to your peers and to a non-technical audience. It takes quite a bit of practice to be able to do this effectively.

We will use a worked example throughout this chapter to illustrate how we go about starting with a research question, developing hypotheses around the research question, presenting statistical results, and creating discussion about the results of our statistical tests. Throughout the worked example, we are using a different data set than in previous chapters but still from the first (1991) wave of the British Household Panel Survey, which can be obtained from the UK Data Archive (www.data-archive.ac.uk).

DECIDING ON A RESEARCH QUESTION

The first thing that you need to do when you are undertaking research is to decide on a feasible research question. The feasibility of a research question depends on many things, including your interests, the time and funding that you have, and your skill set. You may have to narrow a very wide topic to something more specific if you have a limited amount of time in which to produce results. Or you may have to modify a research question if you don't have the analytic skills to answer your original question (provided you don't have the time or desire to learn the new skills whilst answering your research question!).

Suppose you are interested in attitudes towards gender roles. A very broad research question would be, 'What determines attitudes towards gender roles?' But in reality, it is likely that the answer to

this question would require very detailed information about indi
viduals' environments when they were growing up, as well a
detailed information about their parents' beliefs and behaviours
It may be the case that you don't have such detailed information
You may want to narrow your research question to somethin;
more specific, such as, 'How do adults' characteristics influenc
their attitudes about gender roles?'

REVIEWING THE LITERATURE

Before undertaking any study, it important to first review th
existing literature on your general topic. Conducting a literatur
review is beyond the scope of this book, but one of the author
has written about this task elsewhere (see Neuman and Robso
2008). A quick search would show you that Burt and Scot
(2002), Fortin (2005) and McDaniel (2008) have all publishe
studies that examine gender role attitudes. Careful review of thes
articles and others would help you become familiar with theorie
in this area of study and the findings of these studies would assis
you in developing testable hypotheses.

DEVELOPING HYPOTHESES

Hypotheses come from three general places: theory, previou
research, and exploration. Theory and previous research can obvi
ously guide your expectations about what you might find in you
data. In many cases, however, researchers working in new area
may not have previous research or a suitable theory to draw fron
and therefore might undertake exploratory analysis to uncove
patterns in the data. Sometimes scientists use hypotheses that ar
derived from a combination of theory and research, and also hav
additional hypotheses that are exploratory.

From the literature, we would be able to make the followin,
hypotheses:

H1: Women will have more liberal gender role attitudes than
      men.
H2: Younger people will have more liberal gender role attitudes
      than older people.
H3: Married people will have less liberal gender role attitudes
      than other marital statuses.

H4: Religious people will have less liberal gender role attitudes than non-religious people.

H5: Education will be positively associated with liberal gender role attitudes.

H6: Ethnic minorities, particularly Asians, will be less liberal than White respondents.

H7: There will be an interaction between sex and income such that there is a stronger positive association between income and liberal gender role attitudes for women.

We will also include an exploratory hypothesis to test in our analyses:

H8: There will be an interaction between sex and marital status on gender role attitudes.

EXPLORING THE DATA AND SELECTING MEASURES

Our analyses here are going to be based on the same survey that we have been using for the earlier chapters of the book. In 'real life', you may have a choice of data sets from which you could select the data on which you want to test your hypotheses. Or you may have collected your own data for the express purpose of answering a set of research questions.

From the above research questions, we will need measures of: gender role attitudes, sex, age, ethnicity, marital status, religiosity, education, and income.

Recall from Chapter 3 that we constructed a scale that assessed attitudes towards gender roles. After some analysis, it was determined that the following items would be kept in the scale:

opfama: A pre-school child is likely to suffer if his or her mother works.

opfamb: All in all, family life suffers when the woman has a full-time job.

opfamc: A woman and her family would all be happier if she goes out to work.

opfamd: Both the husband and wife should both contribute to the household income.

opfame: Having a full-time job is the best way for a woman to be an independent person.

opfamf: A husband's job is to earn money; a wife's job is to look after the home and family.

opfamh: Employers should make special arrangements to help mothers combine jobs and childcare.

opfami: A single parent can bring up children as well as a couple.

The response categories for all items were: 1, strongly agree; 2, agree; 3, neither agree nor disagree; 4, disagree; and 5, strongly disagree. We reverse coded items *opfamc, opfamd, opfame, opfamh* and *opfami* and then added all the items together to give a scale with a minimum of 8 and a maximum of 40. People who score 8 express very conservative attitudes, while those around the 40 mark would be very liberal. We could have used command **alpha**, but, as shown in Chapter 3, it rescales the variables and their values become less intuitive (although it does produce mathematically the same scale). In this chapter, we will call this variable *genderroles*.

We know from previous chapters that we have a dummy variable that measures sex called *female*, a variable measuring age called *age*, and a marital status variable *mastat*, and a variable that measures monthly income called *fimn*. We also have a seven-category variable that measures education, called *qfachi*, as well as a dummy variable that indicates if a respondent was active in a religious group, which is called *activerel*.

As this example involves adults' characteristics we restrict the sample to those 18 and over.

```
keep if age>17
```

UNIVARIATE ANALYSIS

Before undertaking a detailed analysis, it is important that we get our hands dirty with the data and really get familiar with the variables of interest. All analyses should begin at the univariate (i.e. one-variable) level. We cannot overemphasize that it is important to get to know your variables before you throw them into more complex analyses. In real life, you should also be aware of any sampling issues that are present in your data (i.e. do you need to

include any weights to adjust for sampling?). Don't forget to
specify your missing values!

We can check our variables by running a **summarize** command on our dichotomous and interval variables:

```
su genderroles female age fimn activerel
```

```
. su genderroles female age fimn activerel

    Variable |     Obs        Mean   Std. Dev.    Min       Max
-------------+-------------------------------------------------
 genderroles |    9188    25.50424    4.768196      8        40
      female |    9920     .5333669    .4989106      0         1
         age |    9920    45.49526    18.02041     18        97
        fimn |    9582    758.1702    742.0371       0     11297
    activerel |    9572     .1019641    .3026169      0         1
```

We can see that the mean of *genderroles* is 25.50 with a standard
deviation of 4.77. The sample is about 53% female, and the
average age is 45.50 years. As well, the average monthly income
(*fimn*) is £758.17 and about 10% of the respondents are actively
involved in religious groups (*activerel*).

We will now tabulate the categorical variables in our data set.

```
. ta mastat
```

```
-> tabulation of mastat
```

marital status	Freq.	Percent	Cum.
married	6,009	60.57	60.57
living as couple	670	6.75	67.33
widowed	866	8.73	76.06
divorced	434	4.38	80.43
separated	189	1.91	82.34
never married	1,752	17.66	100.00
Total	9,920	100.00	

We can see that the majority of sample members are married (just
over 60%), with the next largest category being never married
(about 18%).

```
. ta qfachi

highest academic |
   qualification |   Freq.   Percent     Cum.
-----------------+-----------------------------
   higher degree |     122      1.28      1.28
     1st degree |      598      6.25      7.53
hnd,hnc,teaching |     496      5.18     12.71
        a level |    1,349     14.10     26.81
        o level |    2,320     24.25     51.06
            cse |      469      4.90     55.96
  none of these |    4,213     44.04    100.00
-----------------+-----------------------------
          Total |    9,567    100.00
```

The largest category in the variable measuring highest academic qualification (*qfachi*) is 'none of these', which can be interpreted as having only compulsory schooling or less. Just over 7% of the sample had a university degree or higher.

```
. ta race

   ethnic group |
     membership |   Freq.   Percent     Cum.
-----------------+-----------------------------
          white |   9,196     96.15     96.15
    black-carib |      65      0.68     96.83
  black-african |      42      0.44     97.27
    black-other |      26      0.27     97.54
         indian |      99      1.04     98.58
       pakistani |      42      0.44     99.02
    bangladeshi |       6      0.06     99.08
        chinese |       9      0.09     99.17
other ethnic grp |      79      0.83    100.00
-----------------+-----------------------------
          Total |   9,564    100.00
```

In terms of ethnic group membership (*race*), we can see that over 96% of the sample is White. Some of the categories, like 'Black-other', 'Bangladeshi', and 'Chinese', are also very small: 26, 6 and 9, respectively. We need to think if there are ways of collapsing the categories so that we do not have problems with this variable later. If we try to make a number of dummy variables out of this variable the way it is currently coded, we will run into problems with the smaller groups – they will be associated with a lot of 'error' (indicated by large standard errors), or the estimation

echniques will simply kick them out of the estimation procedure
due to collinearity problems.

There are always debates around how to 'best' collapse ethnic
group categories, and there is no one best way. Here, we are going
to group all the 'Black' categories together, create a single group
for Indian, Pakistani, and Bangladeshi called 'Asian', and group
'Chinese' with 'other'. Of course, the Asian group masks the dif-
erences between Muslim and non-Muslim Asians and creating
the single category 'Black' also loses the major cultural differences
between Caribbean Blacks and African Blacks. Also putting
Chinese with 'Other' simply loses the uniqueness of the Chinese in
. very heterogeneous and basically undefined group. But in real-
ife research, such decisions must be made.

```
gen race2=race
recode race2 3=2 4=2 5=3 6=3 7=3 8=4 9=4
.ab def race2 1 "white" 2 "black" 3 "asian" ///
    4 "other"
.ab val race2 race2
```

As a final step, we check our new variable to make sure the
ecoding was done properly.

```
ab race2
```

```
  tab race2

      race2 |    Freq.    Percent      Cum.
------------+-------------------------------
      white |   9,196      96.15      96.15
      black |     133       1.39      97.54
      asian |     147       1.54      99.08
      other |      88       0.92     100.00
------------+-------------------------------
      Total |   9,564     100.00
```

When reading academic articles and reports, the first table that
ou often see is a table of descriptive statistics. It is a good idea to
make such a table to give the reader some indication of the char-
cteristics of your sample. However, notice that in the previous
ables, the N differs quite a bit. For *age* and *female*, there are
0,264 observations, but for *genderroles* there are 9515 and for
ctiverel there are 9902.

Why are the numbers of observations different for the vari
ables? This is due to people not answering survey items. As th
variable *genderroles* is a composite score of eight items, a perso
had to have answered every one of the eight items to be include
in the scale – at least that is how we constructed it here (se
Chapter 3 for alternative techniques that allow for individuals t
be missing on one or more of the items). And some people simpl
don't like to answer certain types of questions, such as those con
cerning income or religious beliefs.

Because of these differing *N* sizes, it is better to wait to pro
duce our final table of descriptive statistics (i.e. the one to includ
in our report) until after we have done our multivariate estima
tions. This is because after we do regressions, we can get th
descriptive statistics for our 'estimation sample' – that is, the sub
sample of cases that have data on all our variables of interest.

We also need to check the distribution of our dependent vari
able so that we know its properties for when we want to conduc
multivariate analyses. We can check this visually with the **his
togram** command.

histogram genderroles, discrete

```
. histogram genderroles, discrete
(start=8, width=1)
```

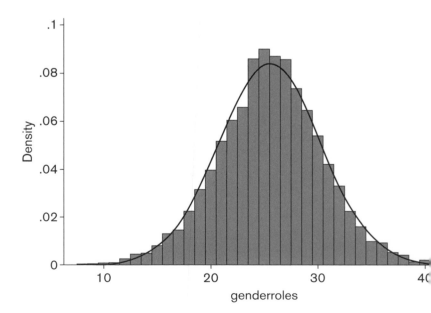

From the histogram we can see that our dependent variable of interest is reasonably normally distributed. It is surprising to see how 'normal' it is, as it is remarkable how few interval variables (in our experience at least) display such tidy distributive characteristics.

BIVARIATE TESTS

Before we directly test our hypotheses, we should undertake some bivariate tests. One of the assumptions of many multivariate techniques is that the independent variables are not highly correlated with one another. We can check this assumption with the **corr** command.

We have two categorical variables in our analysis – *qfachi* and *mastat*. We cannot simply correlate these variables with the others because the numbers associated with their categories are nominal. We need to convert these variables to sets of dummy variables. We can do this with the **xi:** command.

xi: su i.qfachi i.mastat i.race2

```
 xi: su i.qfachi i.mastat i.race2
.qfachi   _Iqfachi_1-7  (naturally coded; _Iqfachi_1 omitted)
.mastat   _Imastat_1-6  (naturally coded; _Imastat_1 omitted)
.race2    _Irace2_1-4   (naturally coded; _Irace2_1 omitted)

 Variable |    Obs       Mean    Std. Dev.   Min    Max
----------+-------------------------------------------------
_Iqfachi_2 |   9567    .0625065    .2420859     0      1
_Iqfachi_3 |   9567    .0518449    .2217253     0      1
_Iqfachi_4 |   9567    .1410055    .3480455     0      1
_Iqfachi_5 |   9567    .2425003    .4286176     0      1
_Iqfachi_6 |   9567    .0490227    .2159267     0      1
----------+-------------------------------------------------
_Iqfachi_7 |   9567    .4403679    .4964572     0      1
_Imastat_2 |   9920    .0675403    .2509681     0      1
_Imastat_3 |   9920    .0872984     .282286     0      1
_Imastat_4 |   9920     .04375    .2045487     0      1
_Imastat_5 |   9920    .0190524    .1367162     0      1
----------+-------------------------------------------------
_Imastat_6 |   9920    .1766129      .38136     0      1
_Irace2_2 |   9564    .0139063    .1171083     0      1
_Irace2_3 |   9564    .0153701    .1230263     0      1
_Irace2_4 |   9564    .0092012    .0954854     0      1
```

You can see that this has created a set of dummies for *qfachi* and *mastat*. This process by default drops the lowest coded variable as the reference category. However, for the **corr** command, we will need all categories for *qfachi*, *mastat*, and *race2* to be dummy coded. We can make the ones corresponding to category 1 for each variable manually. In the case of *mastat*, category 1 corresponds to being married; for *qfachi*, respondents in category 1 have a higher degree; for *race2*, category 1 corresponds to being White.

```
gen married=mastat==1
gen higherdeg=qfachi==1
gen white=race2==1
```

Now we can create a correlation matrix (partial table shown) for all the variables:

corr genderroles age female married _Im* ///
**   higherdeg _Iq* fimn activerel _Irace2* white**

```
. corr genderroles age female married _Im* ///
      higherdeg _Iq* fimn activerel _Irace2* white
(obs=9163)

             | gender~s      age  female married _Imast~2 _Imast~3  _Imast~4
-------------+----------------------------------------------------------------
 genderroles |   1.0000
         age |  -0.3263   1.0000
      female |   0.1472   0.0426   1.0000
     married |  -0.1487   0.1280  -0.0549   1.0000
  _Imastat_2 |   0.1181  -0.1952  -0.0160  -0.3419   1.0000
  _Imastat_3 |  -0.0950   0.4483   0.1626  -0.3749  -0.0815   1.0000
  _Imastat_4 |   0.0410   0.0232   0.0505  -0.2710  -0.0589  -0.0646   1.0000
  _Imastat_5 |   0.0424  -0.0256   0.0472  -0.1760  -0.0383  -0.0420  -0.0301
```

In the correlation matrix, we look for correlations that are higher than about 0.60. We want variables to be correlated with the dependent variable. Because we put *genderroles* first in our list of variables, the correlates with it will be in the first column. What we are trying to spot is if the correlations between our independent variables are of concern. In the full matrix (not presented) we observe that having low education (_Iqfac~7) is quite strongly correlated with *age* (0.4877). Of course, the categories of a variable converted to dummies will be correlated with each other, often quite highly. In this example being *White* and being Asian (_Irace~3) are correlated at −0.6211 (not shown). Apart from these unavoidable correlations between the dummies, there is nothing that raises alarm in this correlation matrix.

If there were a large correlation of, say, 0.70 between *age* and *imn*, for example, we would have to make a decision about dropping one of these variables as multivariate estimation techniques would not be able to properly capture the individual effects of variables that are so highly correlated. Substantively, they are obviously different, but if they are correlated so highly that they are not 'mathematically' different enough for Stata (or any other software program, or even hand calculation for that matter!) to tell them apart.

Note that it was quite 'in fashion' to publish correlation matrices up until about 10 years ago. Now it is very rarely done. If you are writing a technical report, you may want to include such a matrix in an Appendix, but nowadays it is rarely a main part of a scholarly social sciences paper.

We conclude our bivariate tests with some scatterplots.

```
scatter genderroles age, msymbol(point) jitter(3)
```

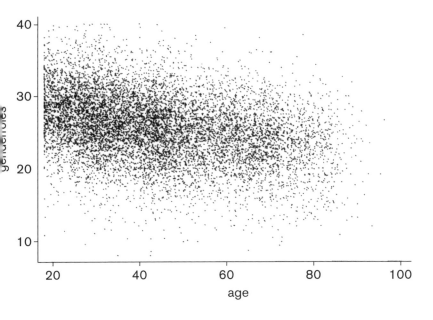

The scatterplot between *genderroles* and *age* reveals that there is evidence of a downward negative linear association. We can also add a linear fit line to display this association:

```
scatter genderroles age, msymbol(point) ///
    jitter(3) || lfit genderroles age
```

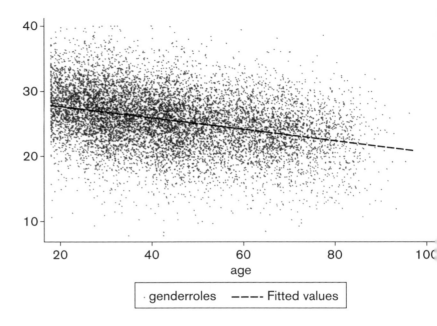

Now we look at the relationship between *genderroles* and total income (*fimn*):

scatter genderroles fimn

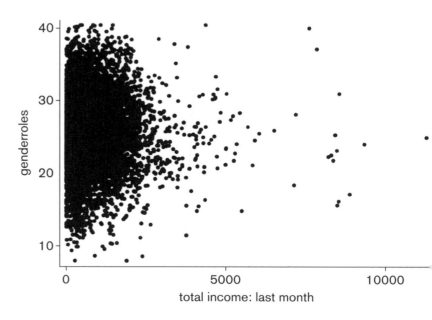

mmediately you can see that the association between these two
variables does not look strongly linear. And there are a number of
outliers – one in particular in excess of £10,000. We need to
examine this income variable more closely.

su fimn, detail

```
. su fimn, detail

                    total income: last month
-----------------------------------------------------------
      Percentiles   Smallest
  1%          0          0
  5%         56          0
 10%     134.23          0   Obs                  9582
 25%     281.45          0   Sum of Wgt.          9582
 50%        550              Mean             758.1702
                 Largest     Std. Dev.        742.0371
 75%    1023.333   8628.875
 90%    1602.562   8716.667   Variance           550619
 95%     2006.54   9455.773   Skewness         3.412333
 99%    3447.667      11297   Kurtosis         27.19502
```

We know that income variables are often highly skewed – and the
details provided from the **su** output reveal this. The mean (758)
and median (550) are very different, and the skewness (3.41) and
kurtosis (27.19) are also very large. In the previous chapter, we
took the natural logarithm of income to help normalize it, as it
was our dependent variable. We could do this, but transforming
income as an independent variable is not often done because it is
not as important when it is an dependent variable. The robustness
of the multivariate tests that are commonly used can cope with
non-normally distributed independent variables.

What we should do, however, is examine what happens if we
eliminate one of the bigger outliers:

corr genderroles fimn

```
. corr genderroles fimn
(obs=9188)

             |  gender~s     fimn
-------------+------------------
 genderroles |   1.0000
        fimn |   0.0278   1.0000
```

corr genderroles fimn if fimn<10000

```
. corr genderroles fimn if fimn<10000
(obs=9187)

             |   gender~s     fimn
-------------+------------------
genderroles  |    1.0000
       fimn  |    0.0282   1.0000
```

The correlations reveal that removal of the outlier only improve
the correlation coefficient by 0.004 – not very much. What if w
limit the sample to those who reported income which was at o
below the 75th percentile?

corr genderroles fimn if fimn<1023

```
. corr genderroles fimn if fimn<1023
(obs=6839)

             |   gender~s     fimn
-------------+------------------
genderroles  |    1.0000
       fimn  |    0.1085   1.0000
```

The correlation on a subsample of those with incomes at or belov
the 75th percentile improves the strength of the association sign
ificantly. So, let's see if we take those below the 95th percentile.

corr genderroles fimn if fimn<2006

```
. corr genderroles fimn if fimn<2006
(obs=8716)

             |   gender~s     fimn
-------------+------------------
genderroles  |    1.0000
       fimn  |    0.0926   1.0000
```

The correlation drops, but only slightly. Therefore, it appears tha
those 472 or so cases with incomes above £2006 per month ar
suppressing the association for the majority of the sample. Ther
are some advanced methods that allow you to model these change
in slopes such as splines, but they are beyond the scope of thi

ook. For this example we will further restrict our sample to those with incomes below the 95th percentile. But before doing this it s worth seeing how many cases will be dropped. We know from the correlations that we will lose about 470 cases who have non-missing values on *genderroles* and *fimn*, but if we use a **keep if fimn<2006** command then we will also drop those missing (.) on *fimn*. Remember that Stata stores missing values (.) as a very large number.

ta fimn if missing(fimn), miss

```
. ta fimn if missing(fimn), miss

   total income: |
     last month |   Freq.    Percent      Cum.
----------------+-----------------------------
              . |     338     100.00    100.00
----------------+-----------------------------
          Total |     338     100.00
```

Or: **count if missing (fimn)**

```
. count if missing(fimn)
338
```

keep if fimn<2006

```
. keep if fimn<2006
(819 observations deleted)
```

This shows us that we had 338 cases missing on *fimn* so when we use the **keep** command we can see that Stata has deleted those plus those under £2006 per month income for a total of 819 cases.

MULTIVARIATE TESTS

As discussed in Chapter 8, there are a multitude of multivariate tests to choose from. You need to pick the one that fits with your hypotheses and the nature of your data. We are testing causal relationships (i.e. that a variety of characteristics influence attitudes about gender roles). Our dependent variable is normally distributed. Therefore ordinary least squares regression is a suitable tool for testing our hypotheses, and we include two interaction terms (Jaccard and Turrisi 2003); see Box 9.1.

Box 9.1: The treatment of dummy variables in interaction terms

We should mention that we have to put **i.** in front of **female** so that Stata knows that it is a categorical variable. However, because dummy variables are a special case of categorical variables (see Chapter 3), if we were interacting two dummies (e.g. *female* and *activerel*), we could just type **i.female*activrel** instead of **i.female*i.activerel**. By way of example, we will show you both ways of doing it.

xi: regress genderroles i.female*i.activerel

```
. xi: regress genderroles i.female*i.activerel
i.female          _Ifemale_0-1    (naturally coded; _Ifemale_0 omitted)
i.activerel       _Iactiverel_0-1 (naturally coded; _Iactiverel_0 omitted)
i.fem-e*i.act~1   _IfemXact_#_#    (coded as above)

      Source |       SS       df       MS              Number of obs =    8712
-------------+------------------------------           F(  3,  8708) =   93.68
       Model |  6160.01762      3   2053.33921          Prob > F      = 0.0000
    Residual |  190871.233   8708   21.9190667          R-squared     = 0.0313
-------------+------------------------------           Adj R-squared = 0.0309
       Total |   197031.25   8711   22.6186718          Root MSE      = 4.6818


------------------------------------------------------------------------------
 genderroles |      Coef.   Std. Err.      t    P>|t|     [95% Conf. Interval]
-------------+----------------------------------------------------------------
   _Ifemale_1 |   1.377705   .1061882    12.97   0.000     1.169551    1.585858
 _Iactivere~1 |  -2.025562   .2970706    -6.82   0.000     -2.60789   -1.443233
 _IfemXact_~1 |   .3858559   .3601664     1.07   0.284    -.3201554    1.091867
        _cons |   24.94691   .0784668   317.93   0.000      24.7931    25.10072
------------------------------------------------------------------------------
```

xi: regress genderroles i.female*activerel

```
. xi: regress genderroles i.female*activerel
i.female          _Ifemale_0-1    (naturally coded; _Ifemale_0 omitted)
i.female*acti~1   _IfemXactiv_#    (coded as above)

      Source |       SS       df       MS              Number of obs =    8712
-------------+------------------------------           F(  3,  8708) =   93.68
       Model |  6160.01762      3   2053.33921          Prob > F      = 0.0000
    Residual |  190871.233   8708   21.9190667          R-squared     = 0.0313
-------------+------------------------------           Adj R-squared = 0.0309
       Total |   197031.25   8711   22.6186718          Root MSE      = 4.6818


------------------------------------------------------------------------------
 genderroles |      Coef.   Std. Err.      t    P>|t|     [95% Conf. Interval]
-------------+----------------------------------------------------------------
   _Ifemale_1 |   1.377705   .1061882    12.97   0.000     1.169551    1.585858
    activerel |  -2.025562   .2970706    -6.82   0.000     -2.60789   -1.443233
 _IfemXacti~1 |   .3858559   .3601664     1.07   0.284    -.3201554    1.091867
        _cons |   24.94691   .0784668   317.93   0.000      24.7931    25.10072
------------------------------------------------------------------------------
```

You can see that the results are identical.

One advantage of using dummy variables as 'interval' variables (as one is essentially doing when dropping the **i.**) is that when you have several interactions with one dummy variable, say *female*, you are not given redundant results.

Suppose we were to interact *female* with marital status, age, and education in our estimation of their impact on *genderroles*.

xi: regress genderroles i.female*age ///
   i.female*i.mastat i.female*i.qfachi

```
. xi: regress genderroles i.female*age ///
>    i.female*i.mastat i.female*i.qfachi
i.female          _Ifemale_0-1         (naturally coded; _Ifemale_0 omitted)
i.female*age      _IfemXage_#          (coded as above)
i.mastat          _Imastat_1-6         (naturally coded; _Imastat_1 omitted)
i.fem-e*i.mas~t   _IfemXmas_#_#        (coded as above)
i.qfachi          _Iqfachi_1-7         (naturally coded; _Iqfachi_7 omitted)
i.fem~e*i.qfa~i   _IfemXqfa_#_#        (coded as above)
```

Source	SS	df	MS
Model	30147.0345	25	1205.88138
Residual	166667.822	8677	19.2080007
Total	196814.856	8702	22.6171979

Number of obs =   8703
F(25, 8677) =   62.78
Prob > F   = 0.0000
R-squared   = 0.1532
Adj R-squared = 0.1507
Root MSE   = 4.3827

genderroles	Coef.	Std. Err.	t	P>|t|	[95% Conf.	Interval]
_Ifemale_1	1.475481	.4216284	3.50	0.000	.6489888	2.301973
age	-.0840634	.0053219	-15.80	0.000	-.0944955	-.0736313
_IfemXage_1	-.0069617	.007236	-0.96	0.336	-.0211461	.0072226
_Ifemale_1	(dropped)					
_Imastat_2	1.736397	.2829492	6.14	0.000	1.181749	2.291045
_Imastat_3	.0771449	.4010154	0.19	0.847	-.7089406	.8632303
_Imastat_4	.9312998	.3949254	2.36	0.018	.1571523	1.705447
_Imastat_5	.3175018	.6461857	0.49	0.623	-.9491755	1.584179
_Imastat_6	.581275	.1986193	2.93	0.003	.191934	.970616
IfemXmas~2	-.7865847	.3891229	-2.02	0.043	-1.549358	-.0238114
IfemXmas~3	.9940145	.4604245	2.16	0.031	.0914732	1.896556
IfemXmas~4	.5622266	.4858379	1.16	0.247	-.390131	1.514584
IfemXmas~5	1.352576	.7614352	1.78	0.076	-.1400176	2.84517
IfemXmas~6	.5004244	.2780129	1.80	0.072	-.0445469	1.045396
_Ifemale_1	(dropped)					
_Iqfachi_1	1.649272	.6709021	2.46	0.014	.3341446	2.964399
_Iqfachi_2	1.199016	.3157355	3.80	0.000	.5800992	1.817932
_Iqfachi_3	-.307903	.3245798	-0.95	0.343	-.9441565	.3283504
_Iqfachi_4	-.2654178	.2197034	-1.21	0.227	-.6960887	.1652531
_Iqfachi_5	-.3738898	.1966644	-1.90	0.057	-.7593987	.011619
_Iqfachi_6	-.858516	.3636598	-2.36	0.018	-1.571376	-.1456564
IfemXqfa~1	.1745363	1.05091	0.17	0.868	-1.885497	2.23457
IfemXqfa~2	-.1261066	.4392844	-0.29	0.774	-.9872082	.734995
IfemXqfa~3	.8151526	.4492686	1.81	0.070	-.0655206	1.695826
IfemXqfa~4	.2182148	.3177161	0.69	0.492	-.4045842	.8410138
IfemXqfa~5	.2559116	.2588053	0.99	0.323	-.2514082	.7632313
IfemXqfa~6	.0685341	.4747771	0.14	0.885	-.8621418	.99921
_cons	28.3311	.3177356	89.17	0.000	27.70826	28.95394

▶

▶   You can see from the output that there are two spaces in the output that say 'dropped'. That is because the main effect of *female* had already been added to the estimation. As there is not a **xi:** option that allows us to specify that the main effects of a categorical variable interacting with a categorical variable (**i.var1*i.var2**) are not reported, we must think of something else.

As dummy variables have some of the 'properties' of interval variables we can use the **xi:** formats **i.var1*var2** as well as **i.var1|var2**. In both of these formats, the second variable is expected to be interval. In the first format, **i.var1*var2**, all interactions as well as the main effects of both variables are reported. In the second format, **i.var1|var2**, all interactions between *var1* (categorical) and *var2* (interval) are created, with the main effects of *var1* not being reported. We can use *female* as our interval variable because it is a dummy and use the **|** option so that Stata doesn't try to enter the main effects of *female* numerous times.

xi: regress genderroles i.female|age ///   i.mastat*female i.qfachi*female

```
. xi: regress genderroles i.female|age ///
>    i.mastat*female i.qfachi*female
i.female         _Ifemale_0-1       (naturally coded; _Ifemale_0 omitted)
i.female|age     _IfemXage_#        (coded as above)
i.mastat         _Imastat_1-6       (naturally coded; _Imastat_1 omitted)
i.mastat*female  _ImasXfemal_#      (coded as above)
i.qfachi         _Iqfachi_1-7       (naturally coded; _Iqfachi_7 omitted)
i.qfachi*female  _IqfaXfemal_#  (coded as above)
```

Source	SS	df	MS
Model	30147.0345	25	1205.88138
Residual	166667.822	8677	19.2080007
Total	196814.856	8702	22.6171979

Number of obs =	8703
F(25, 8677) =	62.78
Prob > F	= 0.0000
R-squared	= 0.1532
Adj R-squared =	0.1507
Root MSE	= 4.3827

genderroles	Coef.	Std. Err.	t	P>|t|	[95% Conf. Interval]	
age	-.0840634	.0053219	-15.80	0.000	-.0944955	-.0736313
_IfemXage_1	-.0069617	.007236	-0.96	0.336	-.0211461	.0072226
_Imastat_2	1.736397	.2829492	6.14	0.000	1.181749	2.291045
_Imastat_3	.0771449	.4010154	0.19	0.847	-.7089406	.8632303
_Imastat_4	.9312998	.3949254	2.36	0.018	.1571523	1.705447
_Imastat_5	.3175018	.6461857	0.49	0.623	-.9491755	1.584179
_Imastat_6	.581275	.1986193	2.93	0.003	.191934	.970616
female	1.475481	.4216284	3.50	0.000	.6489888	2.301973
_ImasXfema~2	-.7865847	.3891229	-2.02	0.043	-1.549358	-.0238114
_ImasXfema~3	.9940145	.4604245	2.16	0.031	.0914732	1.896556

```
_ImasXfema~4 |   .5622266   .4858379    1.16  0.247    -.390131   1.514584
_ImasXfema~5 |   1.352576   .7614352    1.78  0.076   -.1400176    2.84517
_ImasXfema~6 |   .5004244   .2780129    1.80  0.072   -.0445469   1.045396
  _Iqfachi_1 |   1.649272   .6709021    2.46  0.014    .3341446   2.964399
  _Iqfachi_2 |   1.199016   .3157355    3.80  0.000    .5800992   1.817932
  _Iqfachi_3 |   -.307903   .3245798   -0.95  0.343   -.9441565   .3283504
  _Iqfachi_4 |  -.2654178   .2197034   -1.21  0.227   -.6960887   .1652531
  _Iqfachi_5 |  -.3738898   .1966644   -1.90  0.057   -.7593987    .011619
  _Iqfachi_6 |   -.858516   .3636598   -2.36  0.018   -1.571376  -.1456564
 _IqfaXfema~1 |   .1745363    1.05091    0.17  0.868   -1.885497    2.23457
 _IqfaXfema~2 |  -.1261066   .4392844   -0.29  0.774   -.9872082    .734995
 _IqfaXfema~3 |   .8151526   .4492686    1.81  0.070   -.0655206   1.695826
 _IqfaXfema~4 |   .2182148   .3177161    0.69  0.492   -.4045842   .8410138
 _IqfaXfema~5 |   .2559116   .2588053    0.99  0.323   -.2514082   .7632313
 _IqfaXfema~6 |   .0685341   .4747771    0.14  0.885   -.8621418     .99921
        _cons |    28.3311   .3177356   89.17  0.000    27.70826   28.95394
```

You can see here that the results are much tidier, with no 'dropped' messages. This solves the problem of how to tidy up your output with an interaction of a dummy variable with numerous predictors. If the variable you want to interact with numerous other predictors is a categorical variable with numerous categories, however, there is no 'quick fix' to get Stata to stop inserting the main effects several times. There is no 'error' in the results – you will just have to remove the 'dropped' comments manually when you are creating your tables.

To test all of our hypotheses in one model, we can use the command:

```
xi: regress genderroles age i.female*i.mastat ///
    i.qfachi i.female|fimn activerel i.race2
```

```
. xi: regress genderroles age i.female*i.mastat ///
>    i.qfachi i.female|fimn activerel i.race2
i.female          _Ifemale_0-1     (naturally coded; _Ifemale_0 omitted)
i.mastat          _Imastat_1-6     (naturally coded; _Imastat_1 omitted)
i.fem~e*i.mas~t   _IfemXmas_#_#    (coded as above)
i.qfachi          _Iqfachi_1-7     (naturally coded; _Iqfachi_1 omitted)
i.female|fimn     _IfemXfimn_#     (coded as above)
i.race2           _Irace2_1-4      (naturally coded; _Irace2_1 omitted)

      Source |       SS       df       MS              Number of obs =    8692
-------------+------------------------------           F( 24,  8667) =   77.31
       Model |  34656.0981     24  1444.00409           Prob > F      =  0.0000
    Residual |  161881.671   8667  18.677936           R-squared     =  0.1763
-------------+------------------------------           Adj R-squared =  0.1741
       Total |  196537.769   8691  22.6139419           Root MSE      =  4.3218
```

```
----------------------------------------------------------------
genderroles |     Coef.  Std. Err.      t   P>|t|  [95% Conf. Interval
------------+---------------------------------------------------
        age | -.0827785   .0036312  -22.80  0.000  -.0898965  -.075660
  _Ifemale_1 |  .5136454   .1953023    2.63  0.009   .1308066   .896484
  _Imastat_2 |  1.616538   .2740168    5.90  0.000     1.0794   2.15367
  _Imastat_3 |  .0765492   .3888046    0.20  0.844  -.6856002   .838698
  _Imastat_4 |  .9034001   .3914352    2.31  0.021   .1360941   1.67070
  _Imastat_5 |  .2874111   .6373313    0.45  0.652  -.9619098   1.53673
  _Imastat_6 |  .5797909   .1911909    3.03  0.002   .2050114   .954570
_IfemXmas_~2 | -1.063059   .3728356   -2.85  0.004  -1.793905  -.332212
_IfemXmas_~3 |  .8186293    .428668    1.91  0.056  -.0216619    1.6589
_IfemXmas_~4 |  .0240032   .4828787    0.05  0.960  -.9225538   .970560
_IfemXmas_~5 |   .893311   .7512081    1.19  0.234  -.5792355  2.36585
_IfemXmas_~6 |  .2944977   .2572233    1.14  0.252   -.209721   .798716
  _Iqfachi_2 | -.6707918   .5413836   -1.24  0.215  -1.732032   .390448
  _Iqfachi_3 | -1.627406   .5445569   -2.99  0.003  -2.694867  -.559945
  _Iqfachi_4 | -1.673665   .5217301   -3.21  0.001   -2.69638  -.650950
  _Iqfachi_5 | -1.764963   .5151843   -3.43  0.001  -2.774847   .755079
  _Iqfachi_6 | -2.160175   .5498084   -3.93  0.000   -3.23793  1.08241
  _Iqfachi_7 | -1.433279   .5141618   -2.79  0.005  -2.441158   .425399
       fimn |  .0000712   .0001491    0.48  0.633   -.000221   .0003634
_IfemXfimn_1 |  .0019329    .000216    8.95  0.000   .0015094   .0023563
   activerel | -1.305594   .1581752   -8.25  0.000  -1.615655   .9955332
   _Irace2_2 |  1.495979   .4201054    3.56  0.000   .6724727  2.319486
   _Irace2_3 | -1.820171   .3985591   -4.57  0.000  -2.601442  1.038901
   _Irace2_4 | -.6684578   .4874699   -1.37  0.170  -1.624015   .2870991
       _cons |   29.7689   .5729856   51.95  0.000   28.64571  30.89209
----------------------------------------------------------------
```

The information at the top of the output tells us that category 1 in *mastat* has been omitted, as have the categories 1 for *qfachi* and 1 for *race2*. These correspond to being married, having a higher degree, and being White. If the categories that are omitted seem reasonable for testing our hypotheses, you can just leave them. But if it seems more logical to change the reference category, use the **char** command. One of our hypotheses is that education will be positively associated with liberal gender role attitudes, so it probably makes more sense to have the lowest education coded as the reference category, because if support for our hypothesis is found with the default reference category, our coefficients will all be negative – which isn't 'wrong', but less intuitive.

```
char qfachi [omit] 7
xi: regress genderroles age i.female*i.mastat ///
    i.qfachi i.female|fimn activerel i.race2
```

```
char qfachi [omit] 7
xi: regress genderroles age i.female*i.mastat ///
    i.qfachi i.female|fimn activerel i.race2
female          _Ifemale_0-1      (naturally coded; _Ifemale_0 omitted)
mastat          _Imastat_1-6      (naturally coded; _Imastat_1 omitted)
fem-e*i.mas~t   _IfemXmas_#_#     (coded as above)
qfachi          _Iqfachi_1-7      (naturally coded; _Iqfachi_7 omitted)
female|fimn     _IfemXfimn_#      (coded as above)
race2           _Irace2_1-4       (naturally coded; _Irace2_1 omitted)
```

```
  Source |       SS      df         MS              Number of obs =    8692
---------+------------------------------            F( 24,  8667) =   77.31
   Model | 34656.0981    24   1444.00409            Prob > F      =  0.0000
esidual | 161881.671   8667   18.677936            R-squared     =  0.1763
---------+------------------------------            Adj R-squared =  0.1741
   Total | 196537.769   8691   22.6139419           Root MSE      =  4.3218
```

```
------------------------------------------------------------------------------
enderroles |      Coef.   Std. Err.       t    P>|t|     [95% Conf. Interval]
-----------+------------------------------------------------------------------
       age | -.0827785    .0036312   -22.80   0.000    -.0898965   -.0756605
 _Ifemale_1 |  .5136454    .1953023     2.63   0.009     .1308066    .8964842
 _Imastat_2 |  1.616538    .2740168     5.90   0.000      1.0794    2.153676
 _Imastat_3 |  .0765492    .3888046     0.20   0.844    -.6856002    .8386987
 _Imastat_4 |  .9034001    .3914352     2.31   0.021     .1360941    1.670706
 _Imastat_5 |  .2874111    .6373313     0.45   0.652    -.9619098    1.536732
 _Imastat_6 |  .5797909    .1911909     3.03   0.002     .2050114    .9545705
 femXmas_~2 | -1.063059    .3728356    -2.85   0.004    -1.793905   -.3322125
 femXmas_~3 |  .8186293     .428668     1.91   0.056    -.0216619     1.65892
 femXmas_~4 |  .0240032    .4828787     0.05   0.960    -.9225538    .9705602
 femXmas_~5 |   .893311    .7512081     1.19   0.234    -.5792355    2.365857
 femXmas_~6 |  .2944977    .2572233     1.14   0.252     -.209721    .7987164
 _Iqfachi_1 |  1.433279    .5141618     2.79   0.005     .4253994    2.441158
 _Iqfachi_2 |  .7624871    .2247183     3.39   0.001     .3219858    1.202988
 _Iqfachi_3 | -.1941275    .2278045    -0.85   0.394    -.6406785    .2524234
 _Iqfachi_4 | -.2403863    .1581545    -1.52   0.129    -.5504066    .0696341
 _Iqfachi_5 |  -.331684    .1274664    -2.60   0.009    -.5815485   -.0818196
 _Iqfachi_6 | -.7268959    .2308039    -3.15   0.002    -1.179326   -.2744653
       fimn |  .0000712    .0001491     0.48   0.633     -.000221    .0003634
femXfimn_1 |  .0019329     .000216     8.95   0.000     .0015094    .0023563
  activerel | -1.305594    .1581752    -8.25   0.000    -1.615655   -.9955332
  _Irace2_2 |  1.495979    .4201054     3.56   0.000     .6724727    2.319486
  _Irace2_3 | -1.820171    .3985591    -4.57   0.000    -2.601442   -1.038901
  _Irace2_4 | -.6684578    .4874699    -1.37   0.170    -1.624015    .2870991
      _cons |  28.33562    .2710218   104.55   0.000     27.80435    28.86689
------------------------------------------------------------------------------
```

Let's go through the results. We can see from our adjusted R-
uared that our variables explain just over 17% of the variance
gender roles. It isn't brilliant, but it isn't bad either.

We will use $p < 0.05$ to determine statistically significant
ects. In terms of *age*, the effect is statistically significant. Each
ditional year of age reduces a person's score on *genderroles* by −
083, independent of the effects of the other variables. Compared

to males, being female is associated with a 0.514 increase on *genderroles*.

For marital status all the coefficients are relative to the omitte category of married. We need to remember that the Stata-generate dummies for this variable have suffixes that correspond to th original value labels: *_Imastat_2* corresponds to 'living as couple', *_Imastat_3* to 'widowed', *_Imastat_4* to 'divorced *_Imastat_5* to 'separated', and *_Imastat_6* to 'never married Compared to married people, living as a couple was associate with a 1.617 increase in *genderroles*. Being divorced, compared t being married, was associated with a 0.903 increase in *gender roles*. Being single, compared to being married, was also assoc ated with a 0.580 increase in *genderroles*. The other categorie were not significantly different than married at the 0.05 level.

The next lines in our output correspond to the exploratory te of the interaction between sex and marital status. We can see tha three of the interactions are statistically significant. The omitte category here is married males (those who are omitted on bot *female* and *mastat*), so all the results are relative to this grou Significant interactions tell that that the slopes are significantl different for the groups under consideration and cannot be inte preted literally. So the significant interaction between *female* an living as a couple (*_IfemXmas_~2*) means that there is a statisti ally significant difference in the effect of living as a couple o attitudes towards gender roles between men and women. We can be entirely certain of what that difference is without additiona analyses, which we will cover later in this chapter.

In terms of educational attainment, there are four statisticall significant coefficients, which are relevant to the 'none of thes category on *qfachi*, which we interpret as being largely comprise of those with only compulsory schooling. We can see that havin a higher degree (*_Iqfachi_1*) or a university degree (*_Iqfachi_2* compared to having only compulsory schooling, are associate with a 1.433 and 0.762 increase in the *genderroles* measur respectively. The other two statistically significant results are fc having O levels (compulsory school leaving age qualifications) an CSE (Certificate of Secondary Education) relative to having onl compulsory schooling. Both, however, have negative coefficient suggesting that those who have these marginal qualifications a less liberal compared to those with only compulsory schooling (c less). This may have to do with older people being more likely t be in these categories (O levels, for example, have been replace by an alternative qualification). This may be something that esearcher would want to explore in future research. You could create a three way interaction between *age*, *female*, and *qfachi*, dd it to the model and see what happens.

The overall effect of income (*fimn*) was positive and non-ignificant, with each unit (£1) increase in income being associated vith an increase in *genderroles* of 0.00007. This is a very small coefficient, but this is due to the way the variable *fimn* is measured - in pounds.

The interaction between *female* and *fimn* (*_IfemXfimn_1*) was iignificant, though. This suggests that as females earn more, they end to have higher scores on *genderroles*, and that this is iignificantly different from the effect that *fimn* has on males' gender role attitudes. We will explore this interaction in more depth ater in this chapter.

The relationship between being active in a religious group (*activerel*) and *genderroles* is in the expected direction. Compared to respondents who were not active in a religious group, being active in a religious group was associated with a 1.306 decrease in *genderroles*. Finally, in terms of ethnic group membership, we find that relative to Whites, being Black (*_Irace2_2*) is associated with a 1.496 increase in *genderroles*, being Asian (*_Irace2_3*) with a 1.820 decrease in *genderroles* and no significant difference for 'other' (*_Irace2_4*).

Let's review our hypotheses and see what we can determine so far:

H1: Women will have more liberal gender role attitudes than men: supported.

H2: Younger people will have more liberal gender role attitudes than men: supported.

H3: Married people will have less liberal gender role attitudes than other marital statuses: supported.

H4: Religious people will have less liberal gender role attitudes than non-religious people: supported.

H5: Education will be positively associated with liberal gender role attitudes: somewhat supported.

H6: Ethnic minorities, particularly Asians, will be less liberal than White respondents: somewhat supported.

H7: There will be an interaction between sex and income such that there is a stronger positive association between income and liberal gender role attitudes for women: supported.

H8: There will be an interaction between sex and marital status on gender role attitudes: supported.

We have found at least some support for all of our hypotheses. I real life, it is very rare to find support for all your hypotheses Even when you fail to find support for your hypotheses, such 'non-finding' can be a finding in itself (but again, in 'real life' it i actually quite difficult to publish such findings, unfortunately).

If we are satisfied with our models and don't want to make an further adjustments, we can now start thinking about makin, tables and graphs for our paper.

Making tables

Recall that, earlier in the chapter, we urged you to not make table of descriptive statistics until you have run your final model and have an 'estimation sample'. We can get descriptive statistics nov using the **if e(sample)** option or by keeping only the cases in the final regression by using the command **keep if e(sample)** It is very important to note that the following command must b used immediately after the final regression you are using, becaus it is only the last estimates that are stored in memory.

```
gen noqual=qfachi==7
xi: su genderroles age female i.mastat married ///
   i.qfachi noqual fimn activerel i.race2 white if e(sample)
```

```
. gen noqual=qfachi==7
. xi: su genderroles age female i.mastat married ///
>    i.qfachi noqual fimn activerel i.race2 white if e(sample
i.mastat    _Imastat_1-6   (naturally coded; _Imastat_1 omitted
i.qfachi    _Iqfachi_1-7   (naturally coded; _Iqfachi_7 omitted
i.race2     _Irace2_1-4    (naturally coded; _Irace2_1 omitted)
```

Variable	Obs	Mean	Std. Dev.	Min	Max
genderroles	8692	25.54452	4.755412	8	40
age	8692	45.10239	17.99514	18	97
female	8692	.5609756	.4962966	0	1
_Imastat_2	8692	.0700644	.2552702	0	1
_Imastat_3	8692	.0859411	.2802932	0	1
_Imastat_4	8692	.0448688	.2070279	0	1
_Imastat_5	8692	.0196733	.1388828	0	1
_Imastat_6	8692	.1771744	.3818382	0	1
married	8692	.602278	.4894556	0	1
_Iqfachi_1	8692	.0085136	.0918807	0	1

```
-----------+-------------------------------------
_Iqfachi_2 |   8692   .0552232   .2284285   0    1
_Iqfachi_3 |   8692   .0501611   .2182898   0    1
_Iqfachi_4 |   8692   .1390934   .3460639   0    1
_Iqfachi_5 |   8692   .2497699   .4329047   0    1
_Iqfachi_6 |   8692   .0516567   .2213457   0    1
-----------+-------------------------------------
    noqual |   8692   .4455821   .4970585   0    1
      fimn |   8692   649.7487   479.7897   0  2005
  activerel |  8692   .0998619   .2998331   0    1
  _Irace2_2 |  8692   .0125403   .1112854   0    1
  _Irace2_3 |  8692   .0139208   .1171693   0    1
-----------+-------------------------------------
  _Irace2_4 |  8692   .0092039   .0954998   0    1
     white |   8692   .964335    .1854641   0    1
```

ou will notice now that the *N* for all the variables is 8692, which
the same as the *N* for our regression model.

While you can cut and paste the output – as we have done –
to a Word document, it doesn't really resemble a journal-quality
ble. You will have to highlight the table in the Results window
nd then go to **Edit → Copy table**.

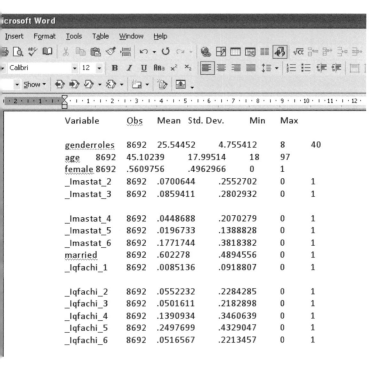

Now open a blank Word document and press **Paste**. The resul[t] will be ugly. Now, in Word, select the contents of the table then g[o] to **Table** → **Convert Text to Table** and the following dialogue bo[x] will appear. More often than not, it is 'smart' enough to guess th[e] number of columns and rows that you want. Check that these ar[e] correct then click **OK**.

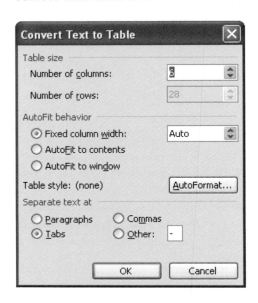

Then you should get this:

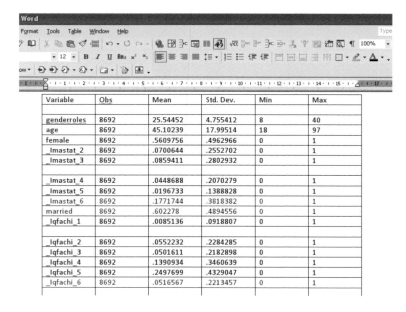

Variable	Obs	Mean	Std. Dev.	Min	Max
genderroles	8692	25.54452	4.755412	8	40
age	8692	45.10239	17.99514	18	97
female	8692	.5609756	.4962966	0	1
_Imastat_2	8692	.0700644	.2552702	0	1
_Imastat_3	8692	.0859411	.2802932	0	1
_Imastat_4	8692	.0448688	.2070279	0	1
_Imastat_5	8692	.0196733	.1388828	0	1
_Imastat_6	8692	.1771744	.3818382	0	1
married	8692	.602278	.4894556	0	1
_Iqfachi_1	8692	.0085136	.0918807	0	1
_Iqfachi_2	8692	.0552232	.2284285	0	1
_Iqfachi_3	8692	.0501611	.2182898	0	1
_Iqfachi_4	8692	.1390934	.3460639	0	1
_Iqfachi_5	8692	.2497699	.4329047	0	1
_Iqfachi_6	8692	.0516567	.2213457	0	1

ome may prefer to copy the table into Excel to do the initial
ormatting rather than Word. With a bit of tidying up, we have
he following table:

able of descriptive statistics (N = 8692)

ariable	Mean	Std. Dev.	Min	Max
Dependent variable				
Gender roles	25.545	4.755	8	40
Independent variables				
Age	45.102	17.995	18	97
Female	0.561	0.496	0	1
Marital status				
Living as a couple	0.070	0.255	0	1
Widowed	0.086	0.280	0	1
Divorced	0.045	0.207	0	1
Separated	0.020	0.139	0	1
Single	0.177	0.382	0	1
Married	0.602	0.489	0	1
Educational attainment				
Higher degree	0.009	0.092	0	1
University degree	0.055	0.228	0	1
HND, HNC, teaching	0.050	0.218	0	1
A levels	0.139	0.346	0	1
O levels	0.250	0.433	0	1
CSE	0.052	0.221	0	1
No qualifications	0.446	0.497	0	1
Income	649.749	479.790	0	2005
Active in religious group	0.100	0.300	0	1
Ethnicity				
Black	0.013	0.111	0	1
Asian	0.014	0.117	0	1
Other	0.009	0.095	0	1
White	0.964	0.185	0	1

The next table you will want to produce is a table of your
regression findings. Let us run the regression again (without displaying the output) to make sure it is the most recent thing in
Stata's memory.

```
xi: regress genderroles age i.female*i.mastat ///
    i.qfachi i.female|fimn activerel i.race2
```

We will now use the command **esttab** to make a regression
table. You might have to install it first. If so, type **findit esttab**

and follow the instructions. There is also a useful online tutorial by the author of **esttab** at http://repec.org/bocode/e/estout/ index.html (Jann 2005, 2007).

If you just type **esttab** after the regression, you will get the following, partial, output in your Results window:

```
_Iqfachi_3              -0.194
                       (-0.85)

_Iqfachi_4              -0.240
                       (-1.52)

_Iqfachi_5              -0.332**
                       (-2.60)

_Iqfachi_6              -0.727**
                       (-3.15)

fimn                 0.0000712
                       (0.48)

_IfemXfimn_1         0.00193***
                       (8.95)

activerel               -1.306***
                       (-8.25)

_Irace2_2               1.496***
                       (3.56)

_Irace2_3               -1.820***
                       (-4.57)

_Irace2_4               -0.668
                       (-1.37)

_cons                   28.34***
                       (104.55)
─────────────────────────────────
N                       8692
─────────────────────────────────
t statistics in parentheses
* p<0.05, ** p<0.01, *** p<0.001
```

As you can see, the results have the unstandardized coefficient and the *t* statistic (in parentheses). At the bottom of the output, there is a note about the *t* statistics being in parentheses and that the stars correspond to * $p<0.05$, ** $p<0.01$, *** $p<0.001$. If you copy this to an Excel spreadsheet, you can edit it from there.

We can tell Stata to make some adjustments to what is displayed. Note that there are far too many options with the **esttab** command to discuss here in any detail. You really need to look at the help menu for this and related commands to truly customize your tables to your liking and to the requirements of specific disciplines and journals.

```
esttab, label se ar2, using regression1.rtf
```

Here, we have requested that variable labels (**label**) be printed instead of the value labels, that the standard errors (**se**) be reported instead of t statistics, and that the adjusted R^2 (**ar2**) is reported. When you use the option **using**, the resulting table is saved as a file in your active directory. Also, when you run the command, a message is returned:

```
esttab, label se ar2, using regression1.rtf
output written to regression1.rtf)
```

The file regression1.rtf is an active link (usually shown in blue) – clicking on it automatically opens up the .rtf (rich text format) document in Word. You should note that you can save the file in many different formats – we are just using .rtf documents to keep things simple. When you click on the active link, your document will open. Again, you will have to tidy it up and add the proper variable names where you used Stata-generated dummy variables. After some tidying up, we have a table that looks like this:

Regression of attitudes towards gender roles on various individual characteristics

	b
Age	−0.0828***
	(0.00363)
Female	0.514**
	(0.195)
Marital status (ref: Married)	
Living as a couple	1.617***
	(0.274)
Widowed	0.0765
	(0.389)
Divorced	0.903*
	(0.391)
Separated	0.287
	(0.637)
Never married, single	0.580**
	(0.191)
Female*Living as a couple	−1.063**
	(0.373)

Female*Widowed	0.819
	(0.429)
Female*Divorced	0.0240
	(0.483)
Female*Separated	0.893
	(0.751)
Female*Never married	0.294
	(0.257)
Educational attainment (ref: No qualifications)	
Higher degree	1.433**
	(0.514)
University degree	0.762***
	(0.225)
HND, HNC, teaching	−0.194
	(0.228)
A levels	−0.240
	(0.158)
O levels	−0.332**
	(0.127)
CSE	−0.727**
	(0.231)
Income	0.000071
	(0.000149
Female*Income	0.00193*
	(0.000216
Active in religious group	−1.306***
	(0.158)
Ethnicity (ref: White)	
Black	1.496***
	(0.420)
Asian	−1.820***
	(0.399)
Other	−0.668
	(0.487)
Constant	28.34***
	(0.271)
Observations	8692
Adjusted R^2	0.174

Standard errors in parentheses
$* \, p < 0.05$, $** \, p < 0.01$, $*** \, p < 0.001$

Understanding interactions

We have two statistically significant interactions: between *female* and a category of *mastat* and between *female* and income (*fimn*). It is often useful, particularly if your audience is non-technical, to give more information about what your interaction means.

Because both of our interactions are with *female*, what the regression coefficients are telling us is that the slopes for males and females on the categorical variables are significantly different from one another. One useful way of getting to the bottom of the interaction is to run the model separately for the variables in the interaction term. So, for example, we can run the models separately for men and women. Instead of just pasting the output for the separate estimations below, we are going to save the results and make a table with both of them using the **estimates store** and **esttab** command.

First, we run a regression for only females (remembering to take out the interactions)

```
xi: regress genderroles age i.mastat ///
    i.qfachi fimn activerel i.race2 if female==1
```

We then get Stata to store these results as a model called 'female'.

```
estimates store female
```

We then run the same model on males:

```
xi: regress genderroles age i.mastat ///
    i.qfachi fimn activerel i.race2 if female==0
```

We store the results as a model called 'male'.

```
estimates store male
```

We then use **esttab** to create a table with results by requesting that models 'female' and 'male' be displayed, with variable labels (**label**), standard errors (**se**), adjusted R^2 (**ar2**), and with only the set of marital status variables (***mastat***) and income (**fimn**) displayed using the **keep** option (as these are the coefficients we are interested in comparing). We write **mtitles** so that each model is given the name we stated above (i.e. 'female' and 'male'). If we don't specify it, the dependent variable would appear

instead. We are using the option **replace** in case we want t
rerun the models for whatever reason. This option overwrites an
existing files with the same name. If we wanted to fix any mistake
and we hadn't written **replace**, Stata would return the followin
message:

```
file interaction.rtf already exists
r(602);
```

esttab female male, label se ar2 ///
  keep(*mastat* fimn) mtitles, ///
  using interaction.rtf, replace

```
. esttab female male, label se ar2 ///
    keep(*mastat* fimn) mtitles, ///
    (using interaction.rtf, replace
 (output written to interaction.rtf)
```

After clicking on the active link, we obtain the following table:

	(1) female	(2) male
mastat==2	0.574* (0.268)	1.566*** (0.277)
mastat==3	0.858*** (0.227)	0.0882 (0.390)
mastat==4	0.890** (0.287)	0.896* (0.385)
mastat==5	1.182** (0.404)	0.262 (0.627)
mastat==6	0.878*** (0.196)	0.537** (0.203)
total income: last month	0.00211*** (0.000177)	0.000000752 (0.000152)
Observations	4876	3816
Adjusted R^2	0.165	0.150

Standard errors in parentheses
* $p < 0.05$, ** $p < 0.01$, *** $p < 0.001$

aphing interactions

eractions presented in a table of regression results are difficult
interpret and not very intuitive. So it is useful to visually display
at they are telling you. Understanding and graphing interaction
ms between a categorical variable and an interval variable is
siderably easier than getting to grips with an interaction
ween two categorical variables. So, we'll start with the inter-
ion between sex and income.

First run the estimation:

```
: regress genderroles age i.female*i.mastat ///
  i.qfachi i.female|fimn activerel i.race2
```

en request predicted/fitted values of *genderroles*:

```
edict xb
```

w we show you two different ways to graph the interaction.
e graphs are slightly different, but both show substantively
t, for women, as income increases so too do their liberal gender
e attitudes, whereas for men there is little, if any, effect, as
wn by the flat line.

First, we graph the predicted values (*xb*) against income
n) separately for males and females, using a linear fit
it) graph. We use a linear fit so that that a single line is
sented. Not using this option and simply requesting a line
ph would result in a crazy looking graph resembling a large
ibble. The **legend** option tells Stata to label the lines as
males' and 'Males'.

```
oway (lfit xb fimn if female==1) ///
  (lfit xb fimn if female==0), ///
  legend(order (1 "Females" 2 "Males"))
```

Alternatively, we could use the **xi3** and **postgr3** com-
ation of commands introduced in Chapter 8. One issue with
s method is that to get accurate predictions of the regression
del a variable can only be in one interaction term. In our
vious model *female* was in two interaction terms so, for this
mple, we remove the **i.female*i.mastat** term and run the

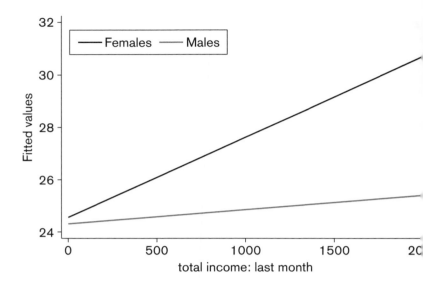

regression model. The **postgr3** command produces the gra
below which tells us pretty much the same as the one above.

```
xi3: regress genderroles age i.mastat ///
     i.qfachi i.female*fimn activerel i.race2
postgr3 fimn,by(female)
```

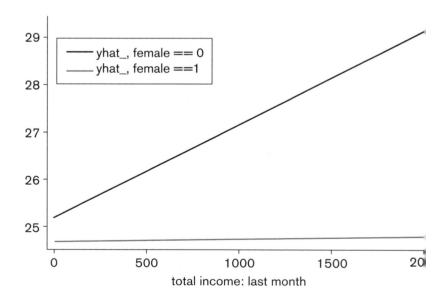

Box 9.2: Doing commands 'quietly'

If you want to rerun a regression just to make sure you have the right estimates in the memory but don't want to see the results you can prefix the command with **qui:** which is short for **quietly**. The **quietly** prefix can be used with commands other than **regress**. You can see from the example command below that it is possible to use the **qui:** prefix before the **xi3:** prefix.

```
qui: xi3: regress genderroles age ///
    i.female*i.mastat i.qfachi fimn activerel ///
    i.race2
```

Recall, from earlier in the chapter, that it was marital status egories 2 (living as a couple), 3 (widowed), and 6 (never mar-d) that were significantly different from 1 (married). We can see m the table on p. 350 that the effect of living as a couple on *iderroles* for males is over twice the size of the effect for nales. Being widowed, on the other hand, has a very large effect women (0.858), but not statistically significant effect for men. nilarly, being separated has a larger effect on women (1.182) in men (0.262).

While the coefficients for these marital statuses look rather ferent for males and females, the lack of their statistical sign-ance in an interaction suggests that their slopes are not nificantly different from one another. This is likely to be due to smaller number of cases when you break down the separated d divorced categories by sex:

mastat sex if e(sample)

```
ta mastat sex if e(sample)
                    |          sex
 marital status |    male   female  |   Total
----------------+---------------------+---------
        married |   2,370    2,865  |   5,235
ving as couple |     292      317  |     609
        widowed |     139      608  |     747
       divorced |     129      261  |     390
      separated |      47      124  |     171
  never married |     839      701  |   1,540
----------------+---------------------+---------
          Total |   3,816    4,876  |   8,692
```

Interactions between dummy coded categorical variables a
quite tricky to understand and even more tricky to present in
meaningful way. This is mainly because the regression coefficier
are not really 'slopes' but differences between groups. An inte
action between a categorical variable and an interval variable,
above, clearly shows a difference in the slopes for the effect
income on gender roles for men and women. Rather than ta
about differences in differences, we shall call the coefficients f
the marital status categories 'slopes', and so we are still looki
for differences in slopes but with the added complication that
the dummy variable coefficients are relative to the same catego
in this case those who are married. Let's look at the relevant pa
of the regression results again:

```
  _Ifemale_1 |   .5136454 .1953023   2.63 0.009   .1308066   .89648
  _Imastat_2 |  1.616538 .2740168   5.90 0.000    1.0794    2.1536
  _Imastat_3 |   .0765492 .3888046   0.20 0.844  -.6856002   .83869
  _Imastat_4 |   .9034001 .3914352   2.31 0.021   .1360941  1.6707
  _Imastat_5 |   .2874111 .6373313   0.45 0.652  -.9619098  1.5367
  _Imastat_6 |   .5797909 .1911909   3.03 0.002   .2050114   .95457
 _IfemXmas_~2 | -1.063059 .3728356  -2.85 0.004  -1.793905 -.33221
 _IfemXmas_~3 |   .8186293  .428668   1.91 0.056  -.0216619  1.658
 _IfemXmas_~4 |   .0240032 .4828787   0.05 0.960  -.9225538  .97056
 _IfemXmas_~5 |    .893311 .7512081   1.19 0.234  -.5792355  2.3658
 _IfemXmas_~6 |   .2944977 .2572233   1.14 0.252   -.209721  .79871
```

We can see that there is a main effect for the *female* variable whe
women, on average, report more liberal attitudes to gender ro
than men. Then three of the marital status categories have sig
ficant main effects in that those living together, those separate
and those who have never been married all have, on average, mc
liberal attitudes to gender roles. The one significant interacti
term between sex and marital status is `_IfemXmas_~2` which
for the 'living together' category. As marital status categories a
dummy coded with married as the reference category, this intera
tion tells us that the 'slope' between 'married' and 'living togethe
categories is different for men and women. None of the oth
interaction terms are significant, which tells us that the 'slop
between those categories and being married is the same for m
and women. These results do not tell us if those who are divorc
are different from those who are separated. This is a drawba
with using dummy coding, and some prefer to use effect codi
to get round this issue of choosing a reference category. S
Chapter 8 for an example of effect coding.

At the risk of being redundant, let's have a look at this using
me graphs. We have done these graphs using the **postgr3**
mmand and then using the Graph Editor to show you what is
ssible in the Editor.

```
postgr3 mastat,by(female)
```

he basic **postgr3** command for the sex and marital status inter-
tion model produces the following line chart. A line chart is not
chnically correct for this, but it gives enough information. In this
aph you can see that the solid line is for women and the dashed
ie is for men. The average difference between these lines repre-
nts the main effect of the female variable, but what the inter-
tion is looking at is the difference in the 'slopes' between each of
e categories and the married categories.

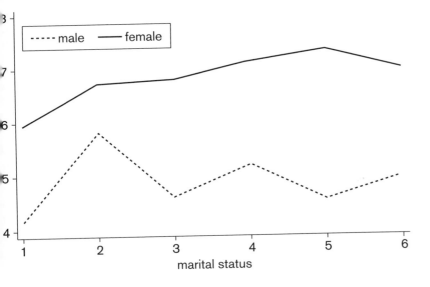

Below we have used the Graph Editor and taken out the lines and
replaced the category points with markers: circles for women and
triangles for men. We have also taken out the information for the
widowed, separated, and divorced categories. To help make our
point three categories are enough. We have plotted the 'slopes'
between the 'married' category and the 'living together' (cohabiting) category with solid lines and between the married category
and the never married (single) category with dashed lines.
Hopefully, this makes it clear that the _IfemXmas_~2 interaction

term is the difference between the two solid line 'slopes'. In oth
words, the difference (slope) between those who are married a
those who are living together is significantly different for men a
women. The difference (slope) is greater for men, which is al
shown by the negative sign on the interaction term's coefficient
the regression results as women are represented by *female=*
Now compare the solid line 'slopes' with the dashed line 'slope
The dashed lines are almost parallel which indicates that there
no gender difference in the differences (slopes) *between tho*
being married and those who have never been married. This
shown in the regression results by the _IfemXmas_~6 interacti
term not being significant. Again, it is worth noting that fro
these results we cannot say anything about differences in 'slop
between other pairs of categories such as between divorced a
widowed. If you wish you can draw in the other three 'slopes' l
tween married and widowed, married and separated, and marri
and divorced for both men and women in the first line graph a
see how they are reasonably parallel, which is reflected in the nc
significant interaction terms _IfemXmas_~3, _IfemXmas_
and _IfemXmas_~5 respectively.

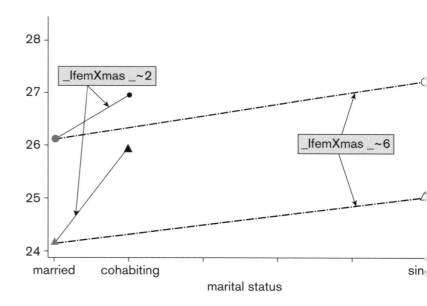

The usefulness of interactions between categorical variables
open to debate. Take this example and ask what this differer
of differences (slopes) actually means. The way we have word

e example, where all categories are relative to those who are
arried, implies what happens when someone changes from that
tegory to another, but is that change logical or the norm? It
ight make a bit more sense to compare those who are living
gether and those who are married with those who have never
en married, as a common social process is from single to cohab-
ng to married. Not all who are married moved from the cohab-
ng or single categories as there will be people who were in the
vorced or widowed categories who then married. However, it
akes little sense to compare those who have never been married
ith those who are separated, divorced or widowed as it is not
ossible to move from being single to being separated, divorced or
idowed without first being married.

WRITING UP YOUR FINDINGS

'typical' research article in the social and behavioural sciences is
rganized in the following way:

.   Introduction
.   Literature review and theory
.   Rationale for current study (highlighting any gaps,
    shortcomings, and/or contradictions in the existing
    literature) and hypotheses
.   Description of data, variables, and analytic approach
.   Results
.   Discussion
.   Conclusion

The best way to learn how to do these steps is to read lots of
articles in your discipline and organize your papers in a similar
way. We've discussed here how to create hypotheses, test them,
understand your output, and make tables and graphs to display
your results. In our opinion, the graphical display of results
is something that is truly underrated in the teaching of social
statistics – and it is a skill that is much appreciated by novices,
policy-makers, and non-technical people who are trying to make
sense of quantitative reports and articles. You should always try
to make complex statistical output as simple to understand as
possible. While you may very much like large tables of numbers
(we sympathize completely), they can be daunting and far from
user-friendly to your proposed readership.

Discussing your results and tying them back in with the lit
ature review is a skill that you can only develop over time. Yo
first attempts are likely to sound like the Results section regur
tated, but it is important to link the findings with previo
research and theory. It is an art, if you don't mind our saying s
This is likely to be the section that you will have to rewrite seve
times. It should also include any shortcomings in your analysis.
you don't acknowledge shortcomings, people reviewing yo
work will be certain to remind you of them. In the example ana
sis undertaken in this chapter, we would be sure to talk about h
the results for education were interesting and unexpected, a
why this might be so (i.e. that older people might be in some of t
classifications). We would also highlight the shortcomings of h
we measured ethnicity and how the results might be maski
important differences between people in the groups. The disc
sion section is also a good place to talk about recommendatio
for future research.

References

Agresti, A. (2007) *An Introduction to Categorical Data Analysis* (2nd edition). Hoboken, NJ: Wiley-Interscience.

Belsley, D.A., Kuh, E. and Welsch, R.E. (2004) *Regression Diagnostics: Identifying Influential Data and Sources of Collinearity*. Hoboken, NJ: Wiley-Interscience.

Berk, R.A. (2003) *Regression Analysis: A Constructive Critique*. Thousand Oaks, CA: Sage.

Bowling, A. (2002) *Research Methods in Health: Investigating Health and Health Services*. Buckingham: Open University Press.

Burt, K.B. and Scott, J. (2002) Parent and adolescent gender role attitudes in 1990s Great Britain. *Sex Roles* 46: 239–245.

Cardinal, R.N. and Aitken, M.R.F. (2006) *ANOVA for the Behavioural Sciences Researcher*. Mahwah, NJ: Erlbaum.

Chen, X., Ender, P., Mitchell, M. and Wells, C. (2003) *Regression with Stata*. www.ats.ucla.edu/stat/stata/webbooks/reg/default.htm.

Fortin, N.M. (2005) Gender role attitudes and the labour-market outcomes of women across OECD countries. *Oxford Review of Economic Policy* 21: 416–438.

Fox, J. (1991) *Regression Diagnostics: An Introduction*. Newbury Park, CA: Sage.

Frankfort-Nachmias, C. and Leon-Guerrero, A. (2000) *Social Statistics for a Diverse Society* (2nd edition). Thousand Oaks, CA: Pine Forge Press.

Frees, E.W. (2004) *Longitudinal and Panel Data: Analysis and Applications in the Social Sciences*. Cambridge: Cambridge University Press.

Goldberg, D.P. and Williams, P. (1988) *A User's Guide to the General Health Questionnaire*. Windsor: NFER-Nelson.

Hinkle, D.E., Wiersma, W. and Jurs, S.G. (1998) *Applied Statistic for the Behavioral Sciences* (4th edition). Boston: Houghton Mifflin.

Jaccard, J. (2001) *Interaction Effects in Logistic Regression* Thousand Oaks, CA: Sage.

Jaccard, J. and Turrisi, R. (2003) *Interaction Effects in Multipl Regression*. Thousand Oaks, CA: Sage.

Jann, B. (2005) Making regression tables from stored estimates *Stata Journal* 5(3): 288–308.

Jann, B. (2007) Making regression tables simplified. *Stata Journa* 7(2): 227–244.

Liebetrau, A.M. (1983) *Measures of Association*. Beverly Hills CA: Sage.

Long, J.S. (1997) *Regression Models for Categorical and Limite Dependent Variables*. Advanced Quantitative Techniques i the Social Sciences, Volume 7. Thousand Oaks, CA: Sage.

Long, J.S. and Freese, J. (2006) *Regression Models for Categorica Dependent Variables Using Stata* (2nd edition). Colleg Station, TX: Stata Press.

McDaniel, A.E. (2008) Measuring gender egalitarianism: The atti tudinal difference between men and women. *Internationa Journal of Sociology* 38: 58–80.

Menard, S. (2002) *Applied Logistic Regression Analysis* (2n edition). Thousand Oaks, CA: Sage.

Mitchell, M.N. (2008) *A Visual Guide to Stata Graphics* (2n edition). College Station, TX: Stata Press.

Neuman, L. and Robson, K. (2008) *The Basics of Social Research Qualitative and Quantitative Approaches* (1st Canadia edition). Toronto: Pearson Education.

Pedhazur, E.J. (1997) *Multiple Regression in Behavioral Research Explanation and Prediction* (3rd edition). Fort Worth, TX Harcourt Brace.

Rabe-Hesketh, S. and Skrondal, A. (2008) *Multilevel an Longitudinal Modeling Using Stata* (2nd edition). Colleg Station, TX: Stata Press.

Rutherford, A. (2001) *Introducing ANOVA and ANCOVA A GLM Approach*. London: Sage.

Ruxton, G.D. and Beauchamp, G. (2008) Time for some a prior thinking about post hoc testing. *Behavioral Ecology* 19 690–693.

inger, J.D. and Willett, J.B. (2003) *Applied Longitudinal Data Analysis: Modeling Change and Event Occurrence.* New York: Oxford University Press.

urner, J.R. and Thayer, J. (2001) *Introduction to Analysis of Variance.* Thousand Oaks, CA: Sage.

Wooldridge, J.M. (2002) *Econometric Analysis of Cross Section and Panel Data.* Cambridge, MA: MIT Press.

Index